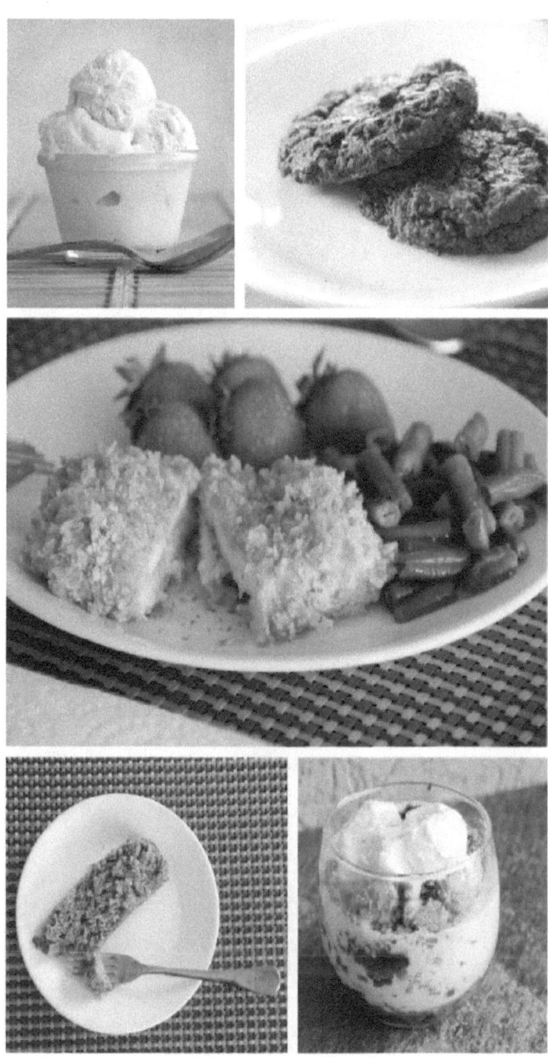

AF583312

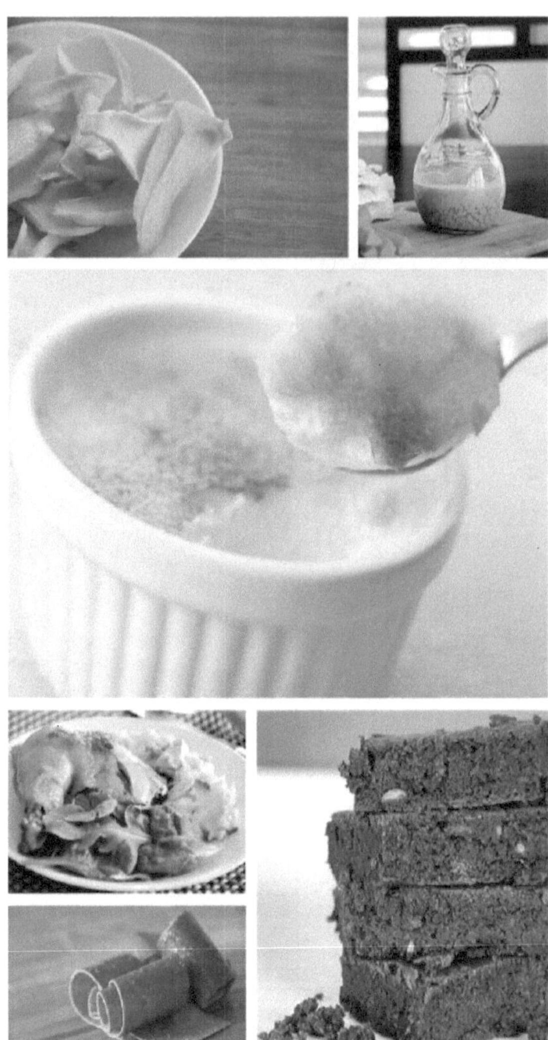

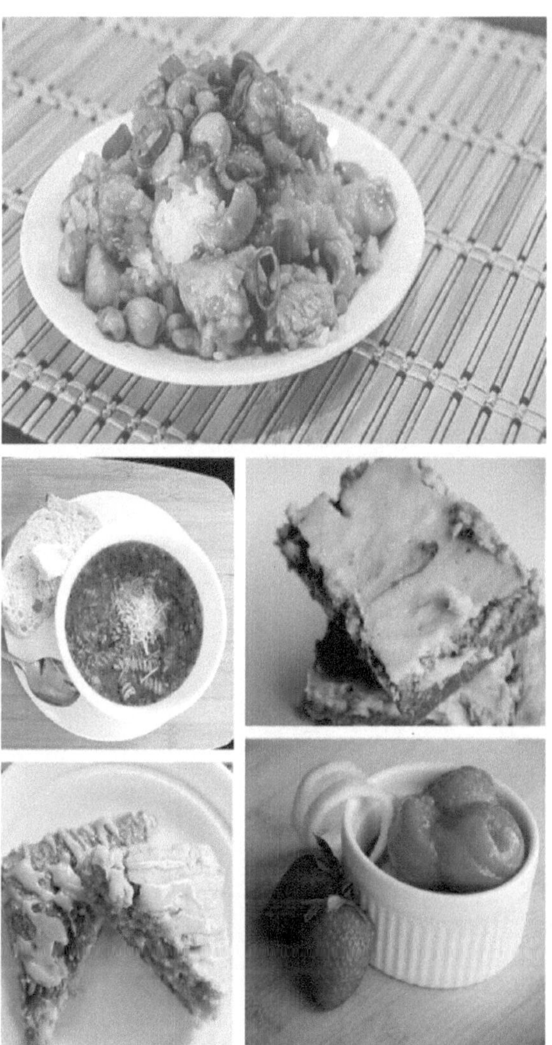

# Table of Contents

SIDE DISHES



SNACKS

DESSERTS

## About this Book

Forget fads and highly restrictive diets. This book is born out of a desire to bring healthy real food (that is also super yummy) to the table... *your table.*

Real food nourishes. It provides energy. It replenishes and repairs cells. It heals.

Those of us who embrace real food say "no" to highly processed ingredients, unnecessary additives, artificial garbage, and other fake food counterfeits. More importantly, however, is that we say "yes" to a variety of different foods. Real food is all around us. It doesn't have to come from exotic places or with a high price tag. A real food diet is a healthy, traditional approach to eating.

**The best part? It's also really delicious.**

Roast chicken, homemade dressings, avocado fries, even dessert… there are lots of comforting and surprising real food recipes within this little book. From sunrise to sunset you will find inspiration in the kitchen that will satisfy the body and soul.

### What is real food?

In a nutshell, here are some of the basics ideas supporting a real food diet:

- Fats, particularly saturated fats are good for you.

- How food was grown and raised matters. Whether one is looking to avoid pesticides, hormones, or animal cruelty, we believe Mother Nature does a better job at food than scientists. Food that is raised naturally not only tastes better, it's better for you.

- Kitchens trump factories and labs.

- There are only 3 macronutrients (carbs, fats, and proteins)… and all are important. I don't push low-carb or low-fat diets. I believe in balance.

- Nutrient density is more important than calorie counting.

- There is no one way to eat healthy. Whether you're primal or vegetarian, gluten-free or a pizza-lovin' fiend… there are many ways to eat healthy and be happy.

# Apple Cinnamon Scones (gluten free)

*By Erica Hale*

**Ingredients:**

2 1/2 cups organic gluten free flour mix (your favorite blend, or try 1 1/2 cups almond meal and 1 cup finely ground coconut flour)

1/2 cup organic, gluten free oats (optional)

1 teaspoon gluten free, aluminum free baking powder

1/2 teaspoon baking soda

1 teaspoon organic ground cinnamon

1 organic, cage free egg

1/2 cup of milk (raw cow's, or coconut or almond milk)

2 teaspoons apple cider vinegar

1 teaspoon vanilla

3 tablespoons organic grade B maple syrup

1 cup grated organic apple (about a whole large apple)

*Optional:* 1/4 cup organic, unbleached evaporated cane sugar, 3 teaspoons ground cinnamon (for sprinkling on top)

**Maple Syrup Glaze**

1 tablespoon coconut oil

1/4 cup organic, grade B maple syrup

1 cup powdered sugar (here's how to make your own!)

**Directions:**

Preheat the oven to 375 degrees.

1. Mix together the dry ingredients.

2. Combine the milk and apple cider vinegar, set aside.

3. Beat the egg, and add the beaten egg, the grated apple, the vanilla, and the maple syrup and mix well.

4. Slowly pour the milk-and-vinegar mixture over the dry ingredients, a little at a time. Watch the consistency of the batter, depending on the juice content of your apple you may need a little more or a little less liquid. You want the batter to be between a very thick cake batter and the kind of cookie dough you drop on the pan.

5. Spread the batter evenly (3/4 inch to 1 inch deep) on a cookie sheet lined with parchment paper, in a roughly rectangular shape.

6. If you want, sprinkle cinnamon sugar over the top.

7. Using an oiled butter knife or pizza wheel, cut through the batter in horizontal lines about 3 inches apart, then vertically to form squares. Cut the squares diagonally to form triangles.

8. Bake for 20 minutes, or until a knife inserted in the center comes out clean.

9. Allow to cool for a few minutes, then pull or cut the scones apart and allow to cool for another 10 minutes.

**For the glaze:**

1. Melt the coconut oil in a pan on the stovetop.

2. Add the maple syrup and powdered sugar, and stir until the glaze is smooth.

3. Drizzle over the scones (make sure they are cool first, or the glaze will melt into the scones) and allow to dry for a few minutes before serving.

# Coconut Flour Pop-Overs

*By Erica Hale*

**Ingredients:**

4 organic, cage-free eggs

1/2 cup milk (grass-fed cow's, coconut, or almond)

3 Tablespoons organic coconut flour (or use almond, rice, wheat etc.)

3 teaspoons organic, grass fed butter (or coconut oil, or omit and use baking cups)

**Directions:**

1. Preheat the oven to 425 degrees.

2. In a muffin tin, place 1/2 teaspoon of butter or coconut oil in each cup. Or, omit and line with baking cups.

3. Melt the butter or oil in the oven until sizzling hot.

4. In a blender or food processor, combine the eggs, milk, and flour. Pulse very well (be sure to pulse one more time before pouring into the pan, to ensure that it's well mixed).

5. Fill each cup 1/2 full with the batter, pouring right over the melted butter or oil.

6. Bake for 20 minutes, until browned on top and cooked through. Don't open the oven door or disturb the pop-overs while they are cooking! The pop-overs will puff up above the pan, but will deflate somewhat as they cool.

Serve hot with your choice of toppings!

*Makes 6 pop-overs.*

# Kale and Mushroom Frittata

*By Erica Hale*

**Ingredients:**

3 cups organic kale, washed and chopped

1/2 a medium-sized organic red onion, thinly sliced

1 cup chopped organic mushroom pieces

2 cloves organic garlic, pressed

1 tablespoon organic coconut oil

6 large, organic cage free eggs

1/4 cup raw organic milk, or cream (coconut milk, rice milk or almond milk also work)

1 teaspoon organic dried dill weed

Sea salt and cracked pepper to taste

**Directions:**

Preheat the oven to 350.

1. Heat the coconut oil in a cast iron skillet. Add the kale and onions, and sauté until they are tender. Add the mushrooms and garlic and sauté a few minutes more. Remove the skillet from the heat.

2. In a bowl, beat the eggs, cream or milk, and herbs. Beat well.

3. Pour the egg mixture over the vegetables in the skillet, do not stir.

4. Place the skillet in the preheated oven, and bake for 20 minutes or until a knife inserted in the center comes out clean.

5. Cut into wedges, garnish, and serve.

*Makes 6 large or 8 small pieces of frittata.*

# Naked Quiche

*By: Robin Konie*

**Ingredients:**

5 eggs (preferably pastured)

2/3 cup whole milk (preferably raw)

1/4 tsp. cayenne pepper

1/4 tsp. paprika

Salt and pepper to taste

1 1/2 – 2 cups chopped veggies (I used tomatoes, bell peppers, green onions, and asparagus, but let your imagination go wild!)

1/2 cup sharp cheddar cheese (or cheese of your choice)

**Directions:**

Preheat oven to 375 degrees, lightly grease a 9″ glass pie pan.

1. Chop veggies into bite small size pieces.
2. In a small bowl, whisk eggs, milk, and spices.
3. Spread chopped veggies across the bottom of the pie pan.
4. Slowly pour egg mixture into pan over vegetables.
5. Sprinkle cheese on top.
6. Bake for 30 – 40 minutes until set. Cool slightly before eating.

## Paleo Pancakes

*By Erica Hale*

**Ingredients:**

2 cups organic, finely ground almond flour

1 cup organic, finely ground coconut flour (or substitute these 2 flours for 3 cups gluten free or whole wheat flour)

6 teaspoons organic, alum free baking soda

3 tablespoons ground organic flax seed

3 cups milk (organic, grass fed raw milk, or coconut milk)

3 tablespoons organic coconut oil (plus more for cooking)

3 free range eggs, separated

*Optional add-ins:*

1 cup mashed banana, applesauce, pear sauce, or pumpkin puree, or one cup organic sour cream or yogurt. (If you are using the add-ins, reduce the amount of milk you use to 2 cups…you may need to add a little more milk if the batter is too thick).

**Directions:**

1. In a large bowl, combine the dry ingredients and mix well.

2. In a second bowl, whip the egg whites until stiff peaks form and set aside.

3. Slowly add the coconut oil, egg yolks, fruit or sour cream/yogurt (if you're using these) and milk to the dry ingredients…beating until well combined after each addition.

4. Fold the egg whites into the batter. If the mixture is thicker than pudding, add a little extra milk.

5. Allow the batter to stand for 20 minutes.

6. In a large skillet, melt some coconut oil to lightly coat the bottom. When the pan is hot (I used medium-high heat on my stove) add the batter…I used 1/3 cup for each pancake.

7. Cook until bubbles start to form and pop, as a general rule when the bubbles don’t refill with batter once they pop the pancakes are ready to be flipped (but, check the first few rounds to make sure this is true for your stove).

8. Flip and cook an additional 1-1 1/2 minutes on the other side.

9. Serve hot with your favorite topping…organic maple syrup, raw honey, or yogurt and fruit!

*Makes 20-30 pancakes.*

# Potato-Crusted Bacon Bits and Egg Pie

*By Eric Hale*

Adapted from: *Cooking for Isaiah*, By Silvana Nardone.

**Ingredients:**

6 slices organic, nitrate-free bacon

2 organic Yukon Gold potatoes, grated and wrung dry

1/2 organic sweet Vidalia onion, chopped (optional)

1 teaspoon paprika

Sea salt and pepper

3 large, organic free range eggs at room temperature, separated

1/2 cup raw organic milk or organic milk substitute (almond, coconut, rice etc.)

1 teaspoon organic yellow mustard

**Directions:**

1. Preheat the oven to 350. In a cast iron skillet or Le Creuset-type baking dish, cook the bacon over medium heat until crispy and the fat has rendered. Remove the bacon and drain on paper towels, leaving the fat in the pan. Allow the bacon to cool, then chop into small pieces.

2. Toss the grated potatoes with the onion (if using), paprika, salt and pepper. Pour into the pan with the bacon drippings and cook without stirring until the bottom of the potatoes is crisp, about 8 minutes.

3. Beat the egg whites until soft peaks form. In a separate bowl, whisk together the egg yolks, milk, mustard and reserved bacon; season with sea salt and pepper and then fold this mixture into the egg whites. Spread over the potato mixture and bake until puffed and golden, about 25 minutes. Let stand for about 5 minutes before slicing.

## Whole Wheat Strawberry Banana Muffins

*By Robin Konie*

**Ingredients:**

2 ripe bananas, mashed

2 eggs

1/4 cup full fat plain yogurt

1/4 cup melted butter or coconut oil

2 Tbs. raw honey

1/2 cup raw organic cane sugar/rapadura

1 1/2 cups freshly ground flour (I've also made them with sprouted flour, too!)

1/2 tsp. baking soda

1/2 tsp. baking powder

2 tsp. pure vanilla extract

1/2 tsp. real sea salt

1 cup fresh strawberries, chopped

**Directions:**

Preheat oven to 350. Line or grease muffin pan.

1. Combine all ingredients, except the strawberries, into your large mixing bowl. Mix on medium-high until smooth.

2. Gently fold in strawberry piece.

3. Fill muffin liners 2/3 full. Bake for 20 – 25 minutes or until a toothpick comes out clean. Let cool on wire rack.

Eat now and freeze and enjoy later!

# SOUPS AND STEWS

# Chicken Noodle Soup from Scratch

*By Erica Hale*

**Ingredients:**

3 organic, free range chicken breasts (skin and bones are OK…whatever you have)

2 quarts water

2 quarts organic, free range chicken stock. Use this recipe, or an organic prepared stock from the store.

3 stalks organic celery, chopped (leaves, too! They add flavor and nutrients.)

3 organic carrots, chopped

1 small organic onion, chopped

4 cloves fresh, organic garlic

2 teaspoons dried organic rubbed sage, or 6 teaspoons chopped fresh sage

1 organic bay leaf

All-natural sea salt, to taste

**Noodles:**

2 cups organic flour, or gluten-free flour substitute. Or use 1 cup coconut flour and 1 cup garbanzo bean or almond flour for grain free.

2 organic, free range eggs

2-4 tablespoons water

**Directions:**

1. In a large stock pot, boil the chicken breasts in 2 quarts of water. When the chicken is done, remove it and allow it to cool enough to remove the skin and bones (if using bone-in) and chop the chicken into very small cubes. Keep the water in the pot boiling.

2. Allow the water to reduce by half as you chop the vegetables and chicken.

3. When the water has reduced, add the chopped vegetables, crushed garlic,

and seasonings as well as the chopped chicken. Pour in the chicken stock and bring back to a boil.

4. Simmer the soup on low for as long as you can, adding water if the level falls below about 3 quarts.

5. Make the noodles (plan to have them ready to add to the soup about 20 minutes before serving):

Pour 2 cups of flour (whichever type you are using) into a bowl. Beat the eggs and drop them onto the flour, mix with a fork until the mixture is combined but dry and crumbly.

Add water, a tablespoon at a time, and stir well. You may use anywhere from one to 4 tablespoons of water, depending on the size of your eggs!

Knead the noodle dough with your hands until it feels elastic enough to roll, but not sticky.

If you are using a noodle maker, roll the dough through one small ball at a time. Fold the dough into a square and then roll it back through the roller, repeat several times until you have a nice, smooth, wide sheet of dough. Repeat with the rest of the dough.

Pass the sheets of dough through the wide noodle cutter, we used a fettuccine cutter.

If you are rolling out the noodles by hand, sprinkle flour onto a clean surface. Roll the dough 1/4 inch thick, and use a pastry cutter to cut wide noodles. Or, use very small cookie cutters (fondant cutters work great) to cut shapes from your dough…or use a pizza wheel to cut noodles the size and shape you'd like!

6. About 20 minutes before dinner, bring the soup to a rolling boil. Drop the finished noodles into the soup a small handful at a time, and cook for 12-15 minutes. If you have extra flour or noodle crumbs left, go ahead and add these too…it thickens the soup a bit and adds flavor!

# Comforting Beef Stew

*By Robin Konie*

**Ingredients:**

2 pounds of stew beef, cut into small pieces

3 Tbsp. coconut oil

4 cups beef stock (chicken stock will also work)

2 cloves of garlic, peeled and left whole

2 bay leaves

2 medium onions, diced

2 tsp real salt

1/2 tsp freshly ground pepper

2 tsp honey

1 tsp paprika

2 dashes of allspice

1/2 tsp ginger

4 tsp balsamic vinegar

2 tsp apple cider vinegar

1/2 tsp cayenne pepper

5 large carrots, chopped

5 ribs of celery, chopped

2 Tbsp. arrowroot powder

**Directions:**

1. Heat oil in a large pot. Brown meat.

2. Add stock, garlic, bay leaves, onions, vinegars, honey, and spices. Bring to a gentle boil and then reduce heat, cover, and let simmer for 1 1/2 hours.

3. Remove garlic cloves and bay leaves. Add carrots and celery. Cover and cook for another 30 – 40 minutes.

4. Remove 2 cups of liquid. Place in a separate bowl. Add arrowroot powder and stir until smooth. Mix back in with the rest of the stew. Stir and cook until hot and bubbly.

*Serves 6 – 8*

## Crock-Pot Chicken Broth

*By Robin Konie*

**Ingredients:**

1 whole pastured chicken (or the frame of a roasted chicken)

1 bag of giblets

3 stalks of celery

2 bay leaves

1 organic onion, cut in half

2 Tbsp. apple cider vinegar

Filtered water

(I leave salt out because it can interfere with the mineral absorption. Just remember to add salt to your recipes as this is a salt-free broth.)

**Directions:**

1. Place chicken or frame, giblets, celery, bay leaves, and onion in large crock pot. Fill with filtered water, leaving 1 inch at the top. Add in vinegar. Let sit at room temperature for 1 hour. (This helps the ACV pull minerals from the bones).

2. Allow the stock to cook for 24 hours on low heat. (Check at 12 hours to make sure water level is still good. Add more water if needed.) If using a whole chicken, you can remove the meat at this point and store for uses in soups, tacos, etc. (The meat is so tender. I just use some tongs and pull it right off the bones).

3. Remove no more than half of the liquid. Strain. Use right away or store. (Chicken stock freezes really well!)

4. Add more filtered water. Repeat step 3: adding water (as needed) every 12 hours, and taking out stock ever 24. You can repeat this for 3 – 5 days. You want a nice rich caramel color. Good broth will become gelatin-like once cooled.

Note: When freezing stock, be sure to leave space in your container for expansion. If using glass, make sure to cool before putting in freezer to keep glass from breaking. You can also freeze stock in ice cube trays… they are the perfect size for making sauces!

## Italian Sausage and Roasted Tomato Soup

*By Robin Konie*

**Ingredients:**

2 Tbs. coconut oil

1 lb. of Italian sausage

1 onion, chopped

4 cloves of garlic, minced

2 tsp dried oregano

1 tsp dried basil

1/4 – 1/2 tsp crushed red pepper flakes

3 – 4 medium sized tomatoes

2 bay leaves

4 cups chicken stock

8 oz. Fusilli pasta

Salt and pepper

Olive oil

Grated Parmesan cheese

**Directions:**

1. Roast the Tomatoes: Cut your tomatoes into small chunks. Spread onto a sheet pan. Drizzle with Olive Oil and sprinkle with Salt and Pepper. Place under your broiler for 5 – 10 minutes, rotating the pan every couple of minutes. (Keep a close eye on these. The skin should start to look wrinkled, but not burned.)

2. While tomatoes are roasting, chop your onion and mince your garlic.

3. Heat coconut oil in large pot over medium heat. Add sausage and stir until it browns, about 5 minutes.

4. Add onions and garlic. Cook until softened, about 4 – 6 minutes.

5. Add spices, roasted tomatoes, bay leaves, and chicken stock. Stir to combine. Bring to a boil and then reduce heat and let simmer for 20 minutes.

6. Add in pasta and cook until al dente, about 10 – 15 minutes. (Be careful not to overcook pasta as it will get mushy).

7. Salt and pepper to taste. Ladle in bowls. Add grated Parmesan cheese on top.

# Parmesan, Zucchini, and Potato Soup

*By Robin Konie*

## Ingredients

2 tablespoon coconut oil

1 medium onion, finely chopped

1 carrot, finely chopped

3 cloves garlic, minced

2-3 medium zucchini, scrubbed but unpeeled, cut into 1/2-inch cubes (about 1 cup)

1 medium russet potato, peeled and cut into 1/2-inch cubes (about 1 cup)

3 cups chicken broth

1 sprig of fresh thyme

1/2 cup milk

1/2 cup sour cream

3 tablespoons freshly grated Parmesan cheese, plus additional for serving

Salt and freshly ground black pepper

Chopped fresh thyme, for garnish

## Directions

1. Heat the oil in a large pot over medium heat. Add the onion, carrot and garlic. Cook, stirring often, until the onions are translucent, about 5 minutes.

2. Stir in the zucchini and potato. Add enough broth to barely cover the vegetables. Add the thyme and bring to a boil over high heat. Reduce the heat to low. Simmer, partially covered, until potatoes are tender, about 15 minutes.

3. Stir in the milk, sour cream, and cheese. Heat until hot, but do not boil. Season to taste with salt and pepper.

4. Ladle into soup bowls, and sprinkle each serving with thyme. Serve hot.

*Makes 4 – 6 servings.*

## Thai Chicken Curry Soup

*By Robin Konie*

**Ingredients:**

3 cups chicken stock or broth

2 2/3 cups unsweetened coconut milk

2 – 3 small hot peppers, seeded and sliced

3 Tbsp. soy sauce (best to get organic to avoid GMOs, preferably naturally fermented)

1/2 tsp ground ginger

2 tsp curry powder

1/4 tsp Real sea salt

1 pound of chicken breasts, thinly sliced

Juice of 1 lime

**Directions:**

1. Bring stock and coconut milk to a boil.

2. Reduce heat and stir in peppers, soy sauce, ginger, curry, and salt. Let soup simmer for 10 minutes.

3. Stir in chicken and limes juice. Continue simmering, stirring occasionally, until chicken is cooked through (about five minutes).

## Winter Vegetable Chowder

*By Erica Hale*

Adapted from *Saving Dinner* by Leanne Ely

**Ingredients:**

3 organic leeks, washed and sliced

1/2 organic onion, chopped

4 slices organic, nitrate-free bacon (optional)

2 large organic russet potatoes, washed and cubed

1 medium butternut squash, peeled and cubed

4 cups organic, free range chicken broth

1/2 teaspoon organic dried thyme

3 cloves organic garlic, pressed

1 cup organic, grass fed raw cream (or 1 cup organic coconut milk)

Real salt and pepper to taste

**Directions:**

1. In a large soup pot, cook the bacon until it's crisp and brown. Remove the bacon and set aside, drain all but about a tablespoon of the bacon drippings.

2. Sauté the leeks in the bacon drippings (omit step one and just sauté the leeks in coconut oil if you'd rather leave the meat out). Add the other chopped vegetables and cook for 3 more minutes.

3. Add the chicken broth or vegetable stock, garlic and thyme, and stir well. Simmer for 20-30 minutes, until the vegetables are soft.

4. Remove half of the vegetables from the soup, and puree in a blender (or mash with a potato masher). Add the cream or coconut milk to the puree, and carefully stir back into the remaining soup.

*Serves 6*

# MAIN DISHES

# Baked Chicken Kiev

*By Robin Konie*

**Ingredients:**

4 chicken breasts, halved

Salt and pepper

2 cups sprouted bread crumbs

1 tsp salt

1 tsp freshly ground pepper

2 eggs

2 tsp water

1/2 cup sprouted wheat flour

Extra Virgin olive oil for drizzling

For the butter filling:

1 cup unsalted butter, room temperature

2 tsp grated lemon zest

1 Tbsp. fresh parsley (or 1 tsp dried)

2 – 4 cloves of garlic, minced

1/2 tsp real salt

1/4 tsp freshly ground black pepper

**Directions:**

1. Prepare butter filling: Using the back of a wooden spoon or a mixer, cream together all the butter ingredients into a small ball. Shape butter into a small 6 x 3″ rectangle on wax paper. Wrap and refrigerate for 2 hours.

2. One at a time, place chicken breasts between two sheets of wax paper. Using a mallet or rolling pin, gently pound the chicken until 1/4 inch thick. Season both sides with salt and pepper.

3. Cut the chilled butter into 8 pieces. Place a piece in the middle of a flattened chicken breast. Wrap chicken around butter, pressing gently to seal any seams. Make sure the butter is completely covered.

4. Combine bread crumbs, 1 tsp salt, and 1 tsp pepper into a small bowl.

5. Whisk 2 eggs with 2 tsp water in a shallow bowl.

6. Spread the flour on a plate.

7. Coat chicken packets in flour, then roll in egg mixture. Finish by coating with bread crumbs, making sure to cover the entire packet. Repeat for all chicken packets and then refrigerate for 1 – 8 hours.

8. Place chicken packets on a greased wire rack on top of a baking sheet. Drizzle chicken with olive oil. Bake for 20 – 30 minutes in a 350 degree oven. Bake until chicken is lightly browned and feels firm when gently pressed.

# Baked Cod with Breaded Parmesan Crust

*By Robin Konie*

**Ingredients:**

2 cups sprouted or sour dough bread crumbs*

2 Tbsp. dried Oregano

2 Tbsp. garlic powder

1/3 cup Parmesan cheese, grated

1 egg

Salt and Pepper

Extra Virgin Olive Oil

4 cod fillets

**Directions:**

Preheat oven to 375 degrees

1. Combine bread crumbs, Parmesan, oregano, and garlic in a shallow bowl.
2. In a separate shallow dish, beat egg with 1 Tbs. of water.
3. Salt and pepper each fish fillet.
4. Coat fillet in egg mixture then in bread crumb mixture.
5. Place breaded fillets on a wire rack on top of a sheet pan. Drizzle each fillet with Extra Virgin Olive Oil. Bake for 15 – 17 minutes or until fish is flaky. Enjoy!

# Carrot Noodles with Peanut Sauce

*By Erica Hale*

**Ingredients:**

10-11 large organic carrots, washed and peeled

2 tablespoons organic sesame oil, divided

1/3 cup organic peanut butter

1 tablespoon apple cider vinegar

3 teaspoons organic maple syrup

1 tablespoon organic soy sauce or liquid aminos

1 tablespoon grated organic ginger root

Red pepper flakes to taste

3-4 cloves organic garlic, pressed

6 organic green onions, washed and chopped

1 cup cooked organic, free range chicken, chopped

Optional: chopped peanuts, bean sprouts, kale, cooked shrimp or crab…you can toss in just about anything, and it's a great way to use leftovers!

**Directions:**

1. Cut the carrots into "noodles" using a vegetable spiralizer, mandolin, or other kitchen tool.

2. Mix together the peanut butter, one tablespoon of the sesame oil, the vinegar, maple syrup, soy sauce, ginger and pepper flakes (if you're using them). If the sauce looks too thick, add a few tablespoons of water and mix well.

3. In a skillet or wok, heat the remaining tablespoon of sesame oil, the garlic, green onions, the chicken and any other ingredients you want to add. Add the noodles and cook until crisp-tender.

3. Pour the peanut sauce over the noodles and stir until combined. Remove from heat and serve.

## Cashew Chicken and Hoisin Sauce

*By Robin Konie*

### Ingredients

2 – 3 large chicken breasts (organic and pastured raised is best), cut into 1 inch cubes

1 Tbsp. arrowroot powder (GMO-free cornstarch can also be used)

Real sea salt and fresh ground pepper

2 Tbsp. expeller pressed coconut oil

6 cloves of garlic, minced

6 – 8 green onions, white and green parts separated, chopped

2 Tbsp. rice vinegar

Hoisin Sauce (see recipe below)

3/4 cups raw cashews, toasted

### Directions

1. Toast the cashews by spreading them on a baking dish and baking for 10 minutes in a 350 degree oven. Place aside.

2. Toss chicken pieces in arrowroot powder and season with salt and pepper.

3. Heat coconut oil in large skillet over medium heat. Cook chicken, garlic, and the white parts of the green onion. Stir often until chicken is cooked through.

4. Add rice vinegar to skillet and cook until evaporated, about 30 seconds.

5. Add homemade hoisin sauce (below) and cook until warm. Add toasted cashews and remaining green onions. Serve over rice, in lettuce wraps, or with any other favorite side.

*Serves 4 – 6*

## Hoisin Sauce

**Ingredients**

4 Tbsp. organic soy sauce (naturally fermented is best)

2 Tbsp. pure peanut butter

1 Tbsp. honey

2 tsp rice vinegar

1 clove of garlic, finely minced

1 tsp hot sauce

1 tsp sesame oil (you can use olive oil in a pinch, but it won't be as "authentic")

Fresh ground pepper

**Directions**

1. Combine all ingredients in a small bowl and whisk to combine.

## Cauliflower Crust Pizza

*By Erica Hale*

**Ingredients:**

3 heads of organic cauliflower, florets cut from stems

1 1/2 cups grated organic, raw milk mozzarella cheese

1 1/2 cups grated organic, raw milk parmesan cheese

3 free range eggs

1 teaspoon crushed organic dry basil

1 teaspoon crushed organic dry oregano

1 teaspoon organic granulated garlic

1 teaspoon sea salt

1/3 cup organic garbanzo bean, coconut or almond flour (or omit and add an extra egg)

**Instructions:**

Preheat oven to 450.

1. Process cauliflower florets in a food processor, pulsing until fine grains form.

2. Place cauliflower grains in a microwave safe bowl, cook for 5- 7 minutes on high (depending on your microwave…look for steam rising from the cauliflower)

3. Spread cauliflower out on a clean dishcloth or cheesecloth and allow it to cool enough to handle. You may need to use 2 cloths for this.

4. Wrapping the dishtowel around the cauliflower, wring out the water as best you can. You might have to work at this for a while, but it's worth it!

5. Put the wrung-out cauliflower into a large bowl, and add the cheeses, eggs, flour (if using) and spices. Mix well.

6. Line several cookie sheets with parchment paper. Pat out the dough in 8-10 inch circles on the paper, about 1/3 of an inch thick. You might want to

create a bit of a lip along the edge of the crust, to better hold in the sauce!

7. Bake the crusts in the oven for 8-10 minutes, until they start to turn golden-brown.

8. Remove from oven, and top with homemade pizza sauce, grated raw milk mozzerella, and whatever all-natural toppings you'd like!

9. Return to oven and bake until the cheese is melted and bubbly.

Enjoy! Store leftover pizza in the fridge, wrapped in parchment paper.

*Makes six 8-10 inch pizza crusts, reducing it by 1/3 would yield 1 roughly 14 inch pizza (or 2 smaller ones).*

## Chicken Fajitas

*By Robin Konie*

**Ingredients:**

1 small onion, sliced thinly

1 red bell pepper, sliced thinly

1 green bell pepper, sliced thinly

1 yellow bell pepper, sliced thinly

1 clove of garlic, minced

2 chicken breasts, sliced thinly

Juicy Chicken Fajitas Marinade:

3 Tbsp. coconut oil, melted

1 Tbsp. extra virgin olive oil

2 Tbsp. lime juice (freshly squeezed is best!)

1 1/2 Tbsp. chili powder

1 tsp oregano

1/2 tsp freshly ground pepper

1/2 tsp real salt

6 – 8 sprouted corn tortillas

Sour cream

Guacamole

**Directions**

1. Combine the onions, peppers, chicken, and garlic in a bowl.

2. In a separate bowl mix all of the marinade ingredients.

3. Pour marinade over vegetables and chicken. Mix well to making sure everything gets coated (I like to put it all in a glass bowl with a lid and then just shake it all up). The coconut oil might "clump" up a bit if the veggies and

chicken are cold. That’s okay. Set aside for an hour (or put in the fridge and let it marinade for a 2 – 8 hours).

4. Heat a frying pan. Add chicken fajitas mixture and sautee for 6 – 10 minutes until the chicken is cooked thoroughly and the onions and peppers are tender.

Serve on tortillas with sour cream, guacamole, and pepper jack cheese. Enjoy!

## Chicken with Lemon Cream Sauce

*By Erica Hale*

**Ingredients:**

Four organic, free range chicken breasts, cut into pieces (2-3 inches).

1/2 cup organic flour (coconut, rice, or wheat all work well)

1 tablespoon organic coconut oil

2 cups organic chicken broth (here's how to make it yourself! Or, substitute 2 cups vegetable broth)

1 cup organic raw cream (or, use 1 cup organic coconut milk)

1/2 cup organic lemon juice

Dash sea salt

**Directions:**

1. Toss the chicken pieces with the flour until they are coated. Save the left over flour (about a tablespoon) for thickening the sauce.

2. Melt the coconut oil in a pan, and add the chicken. Brown the chicken pieces on all sides, and make sure they are cooked through. Remove from the pan and set aside (I put them in a warm oven so they wouldn't get cold).

3. In the same pan that you used for the chicken, add the broth. Scrape the bottom of the pan to incorporate the cooked chicken into the broth. Bring the broth to a boil, and cook until it has reduced by 1/3.

4. Reduce the heat to simmer, then add 3/4 cup of the cream and all of the lemon juice. Stir well.

5. Mix 1 tablespoon of flour into the remaining 1/4 cup of cream, making sure to avoid any lumps. Add this mixture to the sauce and whisk until it's combined, then bring to a boil again and cook until the sauce thickens.

6. Add the cooked chicken back to the sauce, stir to cover the chicken and reheat it a bit.

7. Serve with garlic mashed cauliflower and potatoes and roasted broccoli,

the sauce is wonderful over vegetables!

## Chickpea Nuggets (Falafel) with Cucumber-Yogurt Sauce

*By Erica Hale*

**Ingredients for Chickpea Nuggets:**

1 bag organic, dry chickpeas (soaked overnight, then cooked until soft)

1/3 cup organic extra-virgin olive oil

2 organic, free range eggs

1 Tablespoon organic apple cider vinegar

1-2 cloves garlic (to taste)

2 teaspoons all natural baking powder

1/2 teaspoon sea salt

1/3-1/2 cup flour (chickpea, gluten free, or wheat)

Organic coconut oil for frying

**Ingredients for Cucumber-Yogurt Sauce:**

1/2 large, organic cucumber, peeled

2 cups raw milk yogurt (recipe for homemade)

1 clove garlic

1/4 teaspoon sea salt

1/2 teaspoon dried dill

**Directions for Nuggets:**

1. Place cooked chickpeas into a food processor. Pulse until beans are finely ground.

2. Add the olive oil, eggs, vinegar, sea salt, garlic and baking powder and blend until a smooth paste forms. You may need to add a little water, the mixture should be the consistency of hummus.

3. Transfer the chickpea mixture into a large mixing bowl, and add a little flour at a time until you have a dough that you can work with your hands.

4. Form the dough into nugget-sized pieces, about 1/2 thick and 1 1/2-2 inches long.

5. Fry nuggets in organic coconut oil, you need just enough oil to cover the bottom of the pan (a cast iron skillet works well) and come about 1/2 way up the thickness of the nuggets, about 1/3 in deep. Fry them on one side for about 5 minutes until golden-brown, then flip the nuggets and fry for another 3-5 minutes. Remove the cooked nuggets and allow them to cool for a bit on a plate lined with a paper towel or two.

6. Place extra nuggets on a cookie sheet and freeze until solid, then transfer to a freezer bag for later!

**Directions for Cucumber-Yogurt Sauce:**

Put all the ingredients in a food processor or blender and blend until smooth. Serve with the nuggets for dipping, or serve over gluten free pita bread or naan and vegetables. Store remaining sauce in the fridge.

## Creamy Baked Pasta Rosa

*By Erica Hale*

**Ingredients:**

8 cups dry noodles (shown are brown rice penne noodles, whole wheat also work well)

1 cup raw organic cream

3 tablespoons organic flour (I used rice flour)

6-8 whole organic tomatoes, diced (about 3 cups, include any juice from the tomatoes as well)

3 cloves organic garlic, peeled and pressed

2 teaspoons dried oregano

1 cage-free organic egg, beaten

1 1/2 cups shredded raw, organic mozzarella cheese

1 cup shredded raw, organic Parmesan cheese

Sea salt to taste

Ground black pepper to taste

**Directions:**

1. Start some water boiling in a large pot, and cook the noodles as the package recommends. Start the sauce as the noodles cook.

2. Sauté the diced tomatoes in a cast iron skillet until they are soft and cooked through.

3. In a measuring cup, whisk the flour into the raw cream. Pour over the tomatoes and cook, whisking, continually, until the mixture starts to steam and thicken.

4. Remove from heat, add the garlic and oregano, and salt to taste. Set aside.

5. Drain the cooked noodles and return them to the pot. Toss the beaten egg, 1/2 cup of the mozzarella and 1/2 cup of the Parmesan cheese with the hot noodles (add some ground black pepper if you'd like.)

6. Pour the sauce over the noodles, and stir until combined.

7. Spread the noodle mixture into a large baking dish, and sprinkle the remaining cheeses over the noodles. Bake at 350 degrees for 20 minutes, or until the cheeses are melted and begin to brown.

## Easy Cajun Red Beans with Rice

*By Erica Hale*

**Ingredients:**

32 ounces of dry, organic small red beans (sorted and soaked overnight)

1 large organic onion, chopped

5 cloves of organic garlic, pressed

1 bay leaf

Organic, nitrate free sausage (14 ounces) or 2 organic, free range chicken breasts, finely chopped (meat is optional)

**Cajun Seasoning:**

2 teaspoons sea salt

2 teaspoons organic garlic powder

2 1/2 teaspoons organic paprika

1 teaspoon ground black pepper

1 teaspoon organic ground cayenne pepper

1 1/4 teaspoon organic dried thyme

1 1/4 teaspoon organic dried oregano

Steamed rice of your choice (I like Jasmine rice!)

**Directions:**

1. The night before, sort and soak your beans. Beans should be soaked at least 8 hours.

2. Rinse the beans, and pour them into your slow cooker. Add the chopped onion, garlic, meat (if you're using it) and bay leaf.

3. Combine the spices for the Cajun seasoning in a bowl, mix well. Sprinkle over the beans (I like to use all the seasoning, but you may use less if you like).

4. Cover the beans completely with water, with an extra 1-2 inches of water over the beans (they will swell as they cook, and in the last hours of cooking the water thickens into a broth).

5. Plug in your slow cooker, and let the beans cook on low all day! I allow at least 7-8 hours for cooking.

6. Before dinner, steam or boil the rice of your choice. Stir the beans well, season with extra sea salt to taste, and serve the beans in a bowl over the rice.

Store leftovers in the fridge, or freeze them for a quick meal later! The beans can be thawed overnight in the fridge and reheated on another busy day.

*This recipe makes a lot! It will serve 6 people for 2 meals. Perfect for freezing for later, leftovers, or a large crowd...or cut the recipe in half if you'd like.*

# Easy Crock-Pot Zucchini Lasagna

*By Robin Konie*

**Ingredients:**

3 1/4 cups of quality pasta sauce (or about 26 oz.)

8 ounces organic cream cheese, room temperature

1 container (15 ounces) whole ricotta cheese

Coarse sea salt and ground pepper

2 medium zucchini (8 ounces each), halved lengthwise, then sliced thinly

1 garlic clove, minced

2 teaspoons dried oregano

6 – 8 lasagna noodles

3/4 cup mozzarella cheese

**Directions:**

1. In a small bowl mix the cream cheese and the ricotta cheese. Salt and pepper to taste. (If your cream cheese isn't room temperature, you can always put these ingredients in a small sauce pan and stir over low heat until it's easy to combine.)

2. Mix sliced zucchini with garlic and oregano in a separate small bowl.

3. Pour half of the pasta sauce evenly over the bottom surface of your slow cooker.

4. Place a single layer of lasagna noodles on top of the sauce, carefully breaking pieces as needed to make it "fit" in your slow cooker.

5. Layer half of the cream/ricotta spread over the lasagna noodles followed by a layer of half of the seasoned zucchini.

6. Repeat steps 4 and 5 to create another layer.

7. Finish with a final layer of lasagna noodles. Top that with the remaining pasta sauce. Sprinkle mozzarella cheese on top.

8. Cook on low heat for 4 hours.

# Peanut Chicken Curry

*By Erica Hale*

**Ingredients:**

3 organic, free-range chicken breasts (or omit for vegan…or you can use lamb or beef instead)

4 medium-sized organic russet potatoes, chopped into bite-sized pieces

1 large organic onion, chopped

4 cloves organic garlic, pressed

4 large organic carrots, cut into bite-sized pieces

Feel free to add other vegetables or meat as you'd like…peas, sweet potatoes, kale and cauliflower are all good choices.

**For the Sauce:**

1 cup organic peanut butter. You can also use almond butter.

2 cups organic chicken stock, or vegetable stock

1 cup organic coconut milk

4 tablespoons organic curry powder

1 tablespoon turmeric

1 teaspoon sea salt

1/2 teaspoon cayenne pepper (or more, to taste)

**Directions:**

1. Put the vegetables, garlic and meat into a large pot, or the crockery part of your slow cooker.

2. Mix the spices together.

3. In a separate bowl, combine the spices, peanut butter, chicken or vegetable stock, and coconut milk together until it's smooth.

4. Pour the sauce over the meat and vegetables.

5. Place the pot in the oven and cook at 300 degrees for at least 5 hours. Or, plug in the slow cooker and cook 4-6 hours on high, or 8-10 hours on low.

Speed method (if you really want curry, and you want it now): Heat a little coconut oil in a large cast iron skillet. Cook the chicken until it's done through, then add the vegetables and pour the sauce over it all. Simmer on the stove top until the vegetables are cooked and the sauce is thickened, you may need to add extra chicken or vegetable stock if the liquid boils out before the vegetables are done.

*Serve with cooked basmati rice. Serves six, with possible leftovers.*

# Simple Roast Chicken Recipe

*By Robin Konie*

**Ingredients:**

1 whole chicken, about 4 pounds

1 medium onion, sliced

3 cloves of garlic, peeled

1 lemon, halved

6 – 8 Tbsp. melted butter

1/2 tsp ground thyme

1 tsp ground oregano

Real sea salt

Ground black pepper

**Directions:**

Preheat oven to 375.

1. Spread onions across the bottom of a roasting pan or Dutch oven.

2. Generously salt and pepper the cavity of the bird (make sure to take out any giblets first). Stuff cavity with garlic cloves, 2 Tbsp. of butter, and both halves of the lemon. Place bird upside down on top of onions in pan.

3. Brush outside of bird with 3 Tbsp. of melted butter. Sprinkle oregano, thyme, salt, and pepper over the outside of the bird.

4. Bake in 375 degree oven, uncovered, for 1 hour.

5. Carefully turn bird over, brush again with remaining melted butter and some salt and pepper. Bake for another hour. (If skin starts to get too brown, cover with lid or foil.)

6. After baking, let bird rest for 10 – 15 minutes before moving to a cutting board to carve.

## Savory Stuffed Mushrooms

*By Erica Hale*

**Ingredients:**

20 organic mushrooms

12 ounces organic cream cheese

1 1/2 cup organic Parmesan Cheese, grated and chopped

1 clove organic garlic, pressed

Paprika, for garnish

**Directions**:

1. Wash mushrooms, remove stems and set the caps aside to dry. Finely chop the stems.

2. Soften cream cheese, and add the Parmesan, garlic, and chopped stems. Mix well, then stuff the mushroom caps with the cheese mixture.

3. Arrange mushrooms in a baking dish, and sprinkle with paprika. Bake at 350 degrees until the cheese is brown, bubbly and crispy on top (25-35 minutes, depending on the size of the mushrooms).

# Slow Cooker Chicken Marinara

*By Erica Hale*

**Ingredients:**

2 cans (29 ounces) or two quart jars organic tomato sauce

2 organic zucchini, cubed (add other vegetables to taste)

1 large organic onion, chopped

4-5 cloves organic garlic, pressed

1 Tablespoon organic, dried herbs (basil, oregano, thyme are good options)

2 teaspoons sea salt

3 organic, free range chicken breasts

Organic noodles

**Directions:**

1. In the crockery part of a slow cooker, pour one of the cans/jars of tomato sauce.

2. Layer the zucchini, onion, garlic, spices, and other vegetables (if you'd like) over the tomato sauce. If you're using chicken, put the chicken on top of the vegetables. You can put it in frozen if you'd like.

3. Pour the second can/jar of sauce over everything. Place the crockery in the fridge overnight if you're preparing it ahead.

4. Place the crockery into the electric part of your slow cooker, plug in and allow the sauce to simmer on high for 8 hours.

5. If you have the time, remove the slow cooker's lid for the last 30-40 minutes of cooking. Right before serving, prepare the noodles according to the package. Using a wooden spoon, crush the cooked chicken until it falls apart into tiny pieces.

## Super Easy Honey Mustard Chicken

*By Robin Konie*

**Ingredients:**

4 chicken breasts (preferably organic and humanely raised)

2 Tbs. coconut oil

1/3 cup pure honey

1/3 cup whole grain organic mustard

1 tsp hot sauce (optional)

Sea salt

Fresh ground pepper

**Directions:**

1. Pat chicken breasts with cloth or paper towel so they are dry, and then cut into small strips, sprinkle with salt

2. Whisk honey, mustard, and hot sauce in a small bowl. Salt and pepper to taste.

3. Heat coconut oil in large skillet over medium-high heat

4. Place chicken in heated skillet and cook for 2 – 4 minutes until browned then turn and cook for another 2 – 4 minutes to brown the other side. Depending on the size of your skillet you may need to cook the chicken in two batches so as not to crowd the pan. (It still won't take long, promise.) Once all chicken is lightly browned return everything to the pan.

5. Reduce heat to low. Add sauce to skillet and stir to coat chicken. Heat for a couple of minutes until sauce is warm and chicken is cooked thoroughly.

# SIDE DISHES

# Avocado Fries with Chili Lime Mayonnaise

*By Erica Hale*

**For the Fries**

**Ingredients:**

2 large organic avocados, sliced

1/2 cup milk (organic raw, almond or coconut)

3/4 cups flour (organic gluten free mix, almond, or wheat)

2 large organic, free range eggs

Coconut oil for frying

**Directions:**

1. Heat the coconut oil in a cast-iron skillet (you only need enough oil to cover 1/2 the thickness of the avocado slices).

2. Dip the avocado slices first in the milk, then in the flour, then in the egg, and back in the flour.

3. Carefully place the avocado slices in the oil, and fry until golden brown on one side.

4. Flip the slices over, and fry until the other side is golden brown, too. Remove to a plate covered with paper towels, and repeat until all the slices are fried.

**For the Chili-Lime Mayo:**

**Ingredients:**

1/2 cup mayonnaise (homemade if possible)

1 teaspoon grated organic lime zest

1 tablespoon organic lime juice

1 1/2 teaspoon chili powder

1/2 teaspoon (or to taste) cayenne pepper

**Directions:**

Mix all ingredients together and serve. Refrigerate any unused mayonnaise in an airtight container right away, will keep up to 5 days in the fridge.

## The Best Fruit Salad (with Dairy-Free Option)

*By Robin Konie*

**Ingredients:**

1 12 oz. bag of frozen raspberries (keep frozen- don't thaw)

1 cup of frozen blueberries

2 cups of grapes, halved

4 or 5 kiwi, thinly sliced (or any fruit of your choosing)

1 large lime

3 cans of CHILLED (BPA free) coconut milk OR 16 oz. of heavy whipping cream

1 tablespoon sugar or more to taste (optional)

1 teaspoon vanilla or more to taste (optional)

**Directions:**

1. Whip your coconut milk or heavy cream into a thick cream (see below for coconut cream instructions), adding in vanilla and honey (if so desired).

2. Stir in the juice of the lime and then gently fold in all your fruit.

# Goat Cheese Mini-Tarts

*By Erica Hale*

**Ingredients:**

For the shells:

2 cups of organic almond flour

2 cups grated raw milk sharp cheddar cheese

1 teaspoon dried thyme

6 Tablespoons cold water (I found that I needed closer to 8)

For the filling:

1 organic, cage-free egg

1 tsp. raw milk, organic cream

1/2 cup soft goat's cheese or organic yogurt cheese

1-2 small cloves organic garlic, pressed (optional)

1 teaspoon dried organic parsley flakes (optional)

1/2 cup chopped organic sun dried tomato

1/2 cup chopped organic olives

2 tablespoons chopped organic green onion

1 tablespoon chopped organic fresh basil

**Directions:**

Preheat oven to 300 degrees.

1. In a food processor, blend together the almond flour, cheese, and dried thyme until the mixture looks like course corn meal.

2. Slowly add the cold water, a tablespoon at a time, and watch the dough. When it starts to form a ball, it's ready.

3. Oil a mini-muffin pan well. Press the dough into the muffin cups (about 3 mm thick). Bake at 300 degrees for 20-25 minutes (check for browning at the

edges). Remove from oven.

4. While the tart shells are baking, combine the egg with the cheese, cream, and garlic and parsley (if you're using them).

5. Fill the tart shells with the cheese mixture, then garnish with the chopped sun dried tomatoes, olives, green onions, and basil.

6. Return the tarts to the oven, and bake for an additional 15 minutes (or until the cheese is firm, mine needed 20 minutes).

7. Let cool, and serve!  These are great chilled, too.

## Mango Salsa

*By Robin Konie*

**Ingredients:**

6 roma tomatoes, diced

1 mango, diced

2 cloves of garlic, minced

1/2 bunch of green onions, chopped

1/2 bunch cilantro, chopped

1 jalapeno pepper, diced finely

Real salt and pepper to taste

The juice from one lime

**Directions:**

1. Chop up all ingredients and toss them into a big bowl.
2. Salt and pepper to taste.
3. Drizzle lime juice over the mango salsa, and stir.
4. Eat up!

This mango salsa will stay fresh for a couple of days in the fridge.

## Roasted Radishes and Carrots with Turmeric

*By Erica Hale*

**Ingredients:**

1 1/2 pounds organic radishes, washed with ends trimmed

12 ounces organic baby carrots, washed

2 tablespoons organic grape seed oil (or melted coconut oil)

1/2 of a lemon, juiced

2 teaspoons dried organic parsley flakes

1 teaspoon organic ground turmeric root

1 teaspoon ground black pepper

1/2 teaspoon real salt or sea salt

**Directions:**

Oven 450 degrees

1. Cut your prepared radishes in half, larger radishes may need to be quartered.

2. Place the cut radishes and carrots in a large bowl, and drizzle with the oil and lemon juice. Toss well.

3. Mix the spices together, then sprinkle the mixture over the vegetables and toss until the vegetables are evenly coated.

4. Spread the vegetables out in a single layer on a baking sheet (stoneware works well for this). Roast for 20-25 minutes or until fork-tender (start checking after 15 minutes…mine needed 25 minutes of roasting).

5. Remove from oven, and transfer the radishes and carrots to a serving bowl. Serve right away for the best flavor!

*Makes 8 servings*

## Savory Brussels Sprouts with Pine Nuts

*By Erica Hale*

**Ingredients:**

1 pound organic, fresh Brussels sprouts

1/3 cup organic pine nuts

2 tablespoons organic extra virgin olive oil (or coconut oil)

2 cloves organic garlic, pressed

2 tablespoons balsamic vinegar

3 tablespoons organic cream (may omit)

**Directions:**

1. Wash, trim, and chop the Brussels sprouts. Set aside.

2. In a hot, dry cast iron skillet, roast the pine nuts until they are browned.

3. Add the oil and the Brussels sprouts, cook until the sprouts start to brown and become tender.

4. Add the garlic and balsamic vinegar, stir and cook until the Brussels sprouts are soft and caramelized.

5. Before serving, add the cream and stir, scraping the bottom of the pan, until the flavors are combined.

6. Serve hot, and enjoy!

# Sprouted Wheat (or Spelt) Biscuits

*By Robin Konie*

## Ingredients

2 cups whole wheat (or spelt) sprouted flour

4 teaspoons baking powder (preferably aluminum free)

½ teaspoon real salt

¼ cup cold unsalted butter (preferably grass-fed)

1 cup milk (preferable raw)

## Directions

Preheat oven to 450 and cover a baking sheet with parchment paper (or just grease it). Mix flour, baking powder, and salt in a mixing bowl. (A spoon or a whisk does the job well).

Cut the butter into pea-sized pieces. Cut them into the flour mixture. (You may just end up with pea-sized flour-covered pieces. It will work just fine, though. Promise.)

Pour in milk and gently mix with a spoon until combined. Then give it a couple of more stirs.

Drop by the spoonful onto prepared baking sheet. Gently press down the center of each biscuit slightly with the back of a spoon to ensure that the centers bake through. (You could also shape these and use biscuit cutters, but I would knead the dough a bit first.)

Cook in a 450 degree, preheated oven for 11 – 13 minutes or until golden brown and delicious.

## Sprouted Tortilla Chips fried in Coconut Oil

*By Robin Konie*

**Ingredients:**

Sprouted Tortillas cut into triangle wedges

1/4 – 1/3 cup coconut oil

Sea salt (optional)

**Directions:**

1. Heat coconut oil in a large frying pan over medium/high heat. (I love to use my handy thermometer and start frying once it gets between 300 and 325 degrees.)

2. Place 5 – 7 tortillas wedges in the pan, making sure they don't overlap.

3. Turn wedges over with tongs every 10 – 20 seconds until crisp. (I usually turn mine about four time each… this keeps the edges from burning.)

4. Place on a paper towel or some other cloth to absorb extra oil. Sprinkle with sea salt, if desired.

# SNACKS

# Applesauce

*By Erica Hale*

**Ingredients:**

Apples. That's it! No need to measure them, just use as many as you have... for reference, one quart of sauce will use about three pounds of fresh apples.

**You will also need:**

A large stock pot, a food strainer or food processor, some water, and bags if you are freezing the sauce. If you're canning the sauce, have your usual canning supplies available and freshly sterilized jars, lids and rings.

**Directions:**

Sort the apples. Quarter apples and cut out bad spots. If using a food processor, peel the apples (or, if you don't mind a less smooth texture, leave the skins and process them together).

Put cleaned, quartered apples in a large stock pot. Cover with water, and simmer until apples are soft all the way through.

In small batches, run the apples through a food sieve or food processor until smooth. Repeat until all your apples have been sauced.

If you are freezing the sauce, fill bags the bags with sauce and seal, freeze. If you are canning the sauce, pour out the water from the stock pot and pour the applesauce into the pot. Bring to a simmer and keep hot as you fill your sterilized jars.

Process the jars of applesauce for 15 minutes for pints, 20 for quarts. Don't forget to add extra time if you live at a higher altitude!

## Dark Chocolate Banana Bites

*By Erica Hale*

**Ingredients:**

1 bar (3 ounces) organic, fair trade 65% dark chocolate

2 organic bananas, ripe but firm

**Directions:**

1. Slice the bananas into 1/4 in thick slices.

2. Place the slices on a piece of parchment paper, and freeze them until they are firm (about 1/2 hour).

3. Melt the chocolate gently in a double boiler, or a glass bowl set in a pan of water.

4. Using a toothpick, dip the bananas into the chocolate and place them back onto the parchment paper.

5. Return the chocolate dipped bananas to the freezer, and freeze until the chocolate is set. Transfer them to a container with a lid, and freeze them for snacking later!

## Dried Mangoes

*By Robin Konie*

**Ingredients:**

4 – 5 ripe mangoes

1 Tbsp. raw honey

1/4 cup lemon juice

**Directions:**

1. Mix honey and lemon juice in a small bowl. Stir until the honey is dissolved.

2. Peel and slice mangoes into small even strips.

3. Dip each strip into the lemon/honey mixture, shake off any excess. Place on dehydrator sheets.

4. Dehydrate for 10 – 12 hours at 135 degrees. (I'd start checking around 8 or 9 hours. Times will vary based on humidity levels. Mine took about 11 hours.)

## Gluten-Free Baked Parmesan Crackers

*By Erica Hale*

**Ingredients:**

2 cups of organic flour. You can use gluten free (try 1 cup of chickpea flour and 1 cup of brown rice flour) or grain free (1 cup almond flour, 1 cup chickpea flour) or go with whole wheat flour if you'd like.

1 cup raw milk Parmesan cheese, shredded finely

1/2 cup raw organic milk (you may not need all of it)

1 teaspoon dried organic thyme leaves

Sea salt to taste

Ground black pepper to taste

**Directions:**

1. Place the flour in a food processor or mixer (if using a mixer, make sure your cheese is very finely shredded. A food processor will break the cheese down as it goes, so you don't have to shred it as finely). Add the cheese and the seasonings and blend until combined.

2. Drizzle the milk, a little bit at a time, into the food processor or mixer as it runs. Watch the dough, and stop adding milk when the mixture starts to form a ball and a dry dough is formed.

3. Form the dough into several balls. On a piece of parchment paper, roll out the dough so that it's about 1/8 inch thick. Using a butter knife or a pizza wheel, cut the crackers into squares (or, use a cookie cutter to cut into the desired shape). Poke holes in each cracker with a fork to prevent them from puffing up. Repeat with all the dough.

4. Transfer the crackers, paper and all, to a cookie sheet (no need to grease it first). Bake in a 400 degree oven for 10-15 minutes, or until crisp and browned on the edges.

5. Allow to cool, then break the crackers apart and serve. Store left over crackers in an airtight container.

## Garden Fresh Homemade Guacamole

*By Robin Konie*

**Ingredients**

2 Haas avocados, halved, seeded and peeled

1 lime, juiced

1/2 teaspoon kosher salt

1/2 teaspoon ground cumin

1/4 teaspoon cayenne

1/2 medium onion, diced

2 small tomatoes, seeded and diced

1 small handful of cilantro, chopped

1 clove garlic, minced

**Directions**

1. Scoop out the avocado into a bowl, pour in lime juice, and toss to coat.

2. Drain out the excess lime juice and reserve it for later.

3. Add the salt, cumin, and cayenne and then mash all together using a potato masher.

4. Fold in the onions, tomatoes, cilantro, and garlic. Add 1 tablespoon of the reserved lime juice. Let sit at room temperature for 1 hour and then serve.

# Homemade Granola Bars

*By Erica Hale*

**Ingredients:**

3 cups of organic oatmeal (I used gluten free)

1/2 cup organic peanut butter (or a substitute, like almond butter or sunflower seed butter)

1/2 cup raw honey, or grade B maple syrup, or 1/4 cup of each

1 cup seeds, nuts, or a combination (try pecans, almonds, pumpkin seeds, flax seeds, sunflower seeds, hemp hearts)

1 cup organic, unsweetened and sulfur-free dried fruit (apricots, raisins, cranberries, pumpkin, strawberries, kiwi, dates, figs etc.)

Some good combinations:

Apricot-ginger: 1/2 cup dried apricots, 1/2 cup raisins, 1 tablespoon candied ginger, 1 teaspoon lime zest, 1 cup mixed seeds.

Traditional: 1/2 cup raisins, 1/2 cup golden raisins, 1/2 cup dried cranberries, 1/4 cup sunflower seeds, 1/4 cup almonds.

Tropical: 1/2 cup grated coconut, 1/4 cup dried pineapple, 1/4 cup dried mango, 1/2 cup sunflower seeds, 1/2 cup crushed macadamia nuts, 1/4 cup ground flax seed

Apple-Pie: 1/2 cup chopped dried apple, 1/2 cup raisins, 1/2 cup chopped pecans, 1/4 cup flax seed, 1/4 cup sunflower seeds, 1 teaspoon ground cinnamon.

Dessert bar: 1/2 cup fair trade chocolate chips, 1/2 cup grated coconut, 1/2 cup peanuts, 1/4 cup sunflower seeds, 1/4 cup flax seed.

**Directions:**

1. Pour the oats into a large mixing bowl.

2. Add the fruit, nuts, seeds etc.

3. In a separate bowl, combine the peanut butter (or substitute) and honey.

Mix well, until combined and creamy.

4. Drizzle the peanut butter mixture over the oat mixture, and stir until combined.

5. Line a baking sheet with parchment paper, letting the edges of the paper extend beyond the sides of the pan.

6. Dump the granola mixture onto the parchment lined pan, and press the granola firmly down, in about a 1/2 inch thick layer. Smooth the top.

7. Chill the bars for 1/2 hour in the fridge.

8. Bake bars for 1/2 hour at 200 degrees (this step is optional, but will help your granola bars hold together and be less sticky. You can also cut them and put them in a food dehydrator overnight, or just keep them chilled and eat them raw.)

9. Allow the bars to cool in the pan for 10 minutes, then lift them out using the edges of the parchment paper. Place on a cutting board and cut into bar shapes.

10. Reuse the parchment paper to wrap the finished bars. To keep them fresh, store in an airtight container if you won't be using them soon.

## Homemade Healthy Fruit Snacks

*By Robin Konie*

**Ingredients:**

2/3 cup fresh lemon juice or fresh orange juice (if you don't like sour go with orange!)

2/3 cup frozen or fresh berries (raspberries, blueberries, strawberries are all great.)

1 – 2 Tbsp. honey

5 Tbsp. gelatin (from grass fed cows…)

**Directions:**

1. Pour juice and berries into a small saucepan. Heat over medium heat, stirring occasionally until berries become tender and begin to soften.

2. Add honey and stir until completely incorporated. You will want the fruit to dissolve quite a bit until you have a compote.

3. Puree mixture using a immersion blender or small blender (my magic bullet works great for this!)

4. Let sit, off heat, for 5 – 10 minutes.

5. Whisk in gelatin, one tablespoon at a time. Whisk vigorously until completely incorporated, mixing the gelatin in very gradually to avoid lumps. (If you do get lumps, just run the mixture through your blender again or you can put it back on the heat to help dissolve the gelatin.)

6. Pour into a 8 x 8 or 9 x 9 glass dish. Refrigerate until set (30 minutes to an hour). Cut in small squares. (You could also use some cute molds like this and create awesome shapes. I'm not awesome like that… but you could be!)

Note: I like to keep these in my fridge (I love cold things!), but they do transport and keep nicely at room temperature.

## Juicer Pulp Crackers

*By Erica Hale*

**Ingredients:**

2 1/2 cups juicer pulp

1/2 cup ground organic flax seed

1/2 cup organic, raw sunflower seeds

1 tsp. sea salt

1 tsp. organic dried dill weed

**Directions:**

1. Mix all the ingredients together in a bowl. If your mixture is too crumbly to pat out flat, you may need to add a little water (this might happen if you have a very efficient juicer).

2. Spread the dough onto a Paraflex sheet (if using a dehydrator) or onto parchment paper or foil on a cookie sheet (if you are baking them in the oven). Score the dough into squares with a butter knife or pizza cutter.

3. For a dehydrator, dehydrate at 115 for 2 hours and then break them apart and flip them over, then continue dehydrating for another 2 hours. Check to see if they are crispy, and if they're not ready flip them again and continue to dehydrate for another 15 minutes. Continue to flip and dehydrate every 15 minutes until the crackers are very crispy.

4. For oven dehydrating, set your oven at 150 degrees (or 170 if your oven doesn't go that low). Dehydrate for 1 hour, then check to see if the crackers are crisp. Continue dehydrating, checking ever 1/2 hour, until the crackers are crisp. If you want to omit some of this checking, you can turn off the heat after 2 hours, don't open the oven door and let the crackers sit in the oven overnight.

Dehydrating time will vary quite a bit, depending on how much moisture is in your vegetable pulp, how efficient your food dehydrator is, how low your oven will go, and how humid the air is where you live. It takes some patience the first time you make them, but take notes and the next time you'll know just how long it will take!Store the crackers in an airtight container.

## Juicer Pulp Whipped Cream Cheese

*By Erica Hale*

**Ingredients:**

*For Berry Cream Cheese:*

1 cup organic cream cheese, softened.

1/2 cup berry pulp (blueberries, strawberries, raspberries or a mix of all 3!)

1 tablespoon organic raw honey

*For Vegetable Cream Cheese*:

1 cup organic cream cheese, softened.

1/2 cup vegetable pulp (we like a mix of carrot, onion, tomato, celery and radish…but you can use whatever sounds good!)

1/2 teaspoon sea salt

1/2 teaspoon dried organic dill weed

**Directions:**

If you have a juicer, run the fruit/vegetables through it to juice, and set aside the pulp. If you aren't using a juicer, you can puree the berries in a blender or food processor and finely grate the vegetables or run them through a food processor. Squeeze most of the juice out of the pulp before mixing it in, or the texture of the cream cheese will be too thin.

1. For the berry cream cheese, combine all the ingredients in a mixing bowl and whip, scraping the bowl as needed. Whip until all the ingredients are combined and the texture of the cream cheese is smooth, light and spreadable.

2. For the vegetable cream cheese, combine all the ingredients and proceed as above.

3. Store leftover cream cheese in an airtight container in the fridge for up to 5 days.

## Mango Berry Frozen Yogurt Popsicles

*By Robin Konie*

### Ingredients:

1 ripe mango

5 – 7 medium strawberries (definitely organic)

2 cups full fat yogurt

1/2 tsp vanilla extract

1 – 2 Tbsp. raw honey

### Directions:

1. Mix all ingredients in a blender or food processor

2. Pulse a couple of times (for a chunkier Popsicle) or blend (for a smoother Popsicle) until well combined. (Note: You could stop here and have some the best tasting yogurt on your hands. I won't judge you if you don't make it to the next step.)

3. Pour into Popsicle molds and freeze according to manufacturer's directions. The number of popsicles will depend on the size of your molds.

Viola! Frozen yogurt pops!

# Nacho Cheese Flavored Kale Chips

*By Erica Hale*

**Ingredients:**

2 large bunches organic kale

2 cups organic, raw shelled pumpkin seeds

1 organic red bell pepper, seeded and chopped

1 clove peeled garlic

4 tablespoons fresh squeezed lime juice

1 tablespoon olive oil

4 tablespoons nutritional yeast

1 teaspoon sea salt

½ teaspoon cumin

½ teaspoon turmeric

½ teaspoon onion powder

**Directions:**

Preheat oven to 300 degrees

1. Wash kale well. Tear leaves off of the tough stems, and separate into bite-sized pieces. Spin kale in a salad spinner to dry (or spread it out on a clean dish towel and allow it to air dry).

2. In a food processor, puree pumpkin seeds, bell pepper, and garlic. Add the lime juice, olive oil, yeast and seasonings and puree until creamy. If the mixture is too thick, add water a tablespoon at a time until the mixture is the consistency of thick salad dressing.

3. Toss the pieces of kale with the nacho mixture in a large bowl. Continue to mix until the cheese mixture is evenly distributed on the kale.

4. Cover 3 large cookie sheets with parchment paper. Arrange the kale in a single layer on the paper, being careful not to let the pieces overlap.

5. Bake in the oven at 300 degrees for 10 minutes, then flip them and bake another 10 minutes. Turn off oven and allow to rest for several hours, until completely dry. Or, place on trays in a food dehydrator and dehydrate on low for 10 hours.

Store these in an airtight container or large zip lock bag, and enjoy guilt-free snacking!

## Roasted Chickpea Snacks (in 3 flavors)

*By Erica Hale*

**Ingredients:**

1 16 ounce bag organic chickpeas (garbanzo beans), soaked overnight

**For BBQ seasoning** (each seasoning mix covers 1/3 of the beans):

2 Tbsp. organic extra virgin olive oil

2 tsp. chili powder

2 tsp. organic apple cider vinegar

2 tsp. organic rapadura or organic cane sugar

1 tsp. paprika

1 tsp. cumin

1 tsp. organic, stone ground mustard

1 tsp. garlic powder

1 tsp. onion powder

1 tsp. sea salt

**For Salt and Vinegar seasoning**

2 cups organic white vinegar

1 tbsp. sea salt

2 tsp. organic extra-virgin olive oil

**For Chili-Lime seasoning**

2 tsp. organic extra-virgin olive oil

2 tsp. chili powder

2 tsp. zest from an organic lime

2 tsp. finely grated ginger root

1 tsp. sea salt

**Directions:**

Preheat oven to 400 degrees.

Prepare the beans: Cover the soaked beans with water (you want about twice the amount of water as beans), boil until soft, about an hour. Drain and rinse beans, allow to dry in a collander.

For Salt and Vinegar flavor: Place 1/3 of the beans in a sauce pan, and pour 2 cups of vinegar over them. Boil the beans in vinegar for 1/2 hour, drain and do not rinse. Toss beans with sea salt and olive oil, making sure they are evenly coated. Pour beans on an oiled cookie sheet in a single layer.

For BBQ and Chili-Lime flavors: Mix all ingredients for BBQ flavor together in a bowl. Add 1/3 of the prepared beans to the bowl, and stir until the beans are well coated. Pour beans onto a greased cookie sheet, making sure that they are in a single layer. Repeat with Chili-Lime ingredients, and another 1/3 of the beans.

Roast the chickpeas in the oven for 30-40 minutes, watching them so that they don't burn. You will want to start checking them after about 25 minutes, as they will quickly go from nicely browned to too brown!

Store in an airtight container.

## Raspberry Yogurt Fruit Leather

*By Robin Konie*

**Ingredients:**

1 cup fresh or frozen raspberries (preferably organic as berries are high in pesticides)

2 cups full fat yogurt (recipe to make your own)

1 tsp vanilla extract

1 – 2 Tbsp. honey

**Directions:**

1. Put all ingredients in a blender or food processor. Blend until smooth.

2. Cover your dehydrator trays with plastic wrap or unbleached parchment paper.

3. Spread the yogurt mixture thinly over 2 – 3 trays. (Mine took up two trays in my Excaliber Dehydrator.)

4. Dehydrate at 135 degrees for 6 – 8 hours (I'd start checking around 4 hours, as humidity levels will change the time for everyone. Mine took about 7 hours.)

5. Cut up in strips and store in an air tight container.

# DESSERTS

# 3 Ingredient Peanut Butter Cookies

*By Erica Hale*

**Ingredients:**

1 organic, cage-free egg

1 cup organic peanut butter (or almond butter)

1/3 cup organic honey

Optional: organic fair-trade chocolate chips (1/2 cup), or organic raisins (1/2 cup), or 1/4 cup shredded coconut and 1/4 cup pitted dates, or 1/4 cup chopped dried fruit and 1/4 cup nuts…or you choose what to put in!

**Directions:**

Oven 350

1. Mix all the ingredients together, stirring well.

2. Line a cookie sheet with parchment paper. Drop the batter on the paper, a heaping tablespoon for each cookie.

3. Bake for 8 minutes. Cookies should start to brown slightly around the edges. They may seem too soft, but if they're starting to brown they're good to go!

4. Let the cookies cool for 5 minutes (they will firm up as they cool).

*Makes 18-24 cookies*

# Avocado Chocolate Cookies

*By Erica Hale*

**Ingredients:**

4 ounces organic, fair trade unsweetened chocolate melted in 1 tbsp. coconut oil

1 organic avocado

1/4 cup unsalted organic almond butter (may substitute peanut butter)

1/2 cup honey

3 organic, cage-free eggs

1/4 cup organic cocoa powder

3 tbsp. organic almond flour

**Instructions:**

1. In a food processor, puree the avocado until it's very smooth.

2. Add the other ingredients, one ingredient at a time, and pulse until the batter is combined.

3. Chill the batter in the fridge for at least an hour.

4. Fill a pastry bag with the chilled batter and pipe the batter out onto a cookie sheet lined with parchment paper, about a tablespoon at a time. Or, drop the chilled batter onto the paper by heaping tablespoonful.

5. Bake at 350 degrees for 15-17 minutes (check after 15 minutes).

6. Allow the cookies to cool for five minutes, then remove to a cooling rack or plate.

Enjoy!

# Black Bean Brownies

*By Robin Konie*

**Ingredients**

1 can black beans (BPA free), drained and rinsed

2 eggs

2 – 3 Tbsp. of peanut butter (optional, but adds a fun flavor)

4 Tbsp. coconut oil

4 Tbsp. cocoa powder (unsweetened)

1 tsp vanilla

3/4 cup organic cane sugar

1/2 tsp real salt

1/4 cup rolled oats (optional)

**Directions:**

Preheat oven to 350°

1. Pour drained beans into a blender or food processor, blend until smooth.

2. Add the remaining ingredients, except the oats, and continue blending until evenly mixed.

3. Stir in the oats, if using.

4. Pour mixture into a greased 8 x 8 pan. Bake for about 30 minutes or until a toothpick comes out clean.

5. Cool and Enjoy!

## Cast Iron Sprouted Berry Cobbler

*By Robin Konie*

**Ingredients:**

1 1/2 cups sprouted wheat or spelt flour

1 cup rapadura or organic cane sugar

3 Tbs. raw honey

1/2 tsp real sea salt

2 1/2 tsp aluminum free baking powder

1 1/2 cup whole milk (raw and organic, if you please)

1/2 cup (1 stick) butter

3 cups of fresh or frozen berries, divided (strawberries, raspberries, blackberries, and blueberries are all good. Cut any larger berries into bite size pieces.)

Juice of 1 lemon

**Directions:**

Preheat oven to 350 degrees

1. In your cast iron skillet (12″), heat over medium-high heat 1 1/2 cups of berries, honey, and lemon juice. Stir for 10 or so minutes until berries begin to break down into a thick compote. Pour mixture into a bowl and add the remaining uncooked berries. Mix together and let cool slightly.

2. Add butter to the now empty cast iron skillet and let melt completely.

3. Meanwhile, in a separate bowl whisk flour, sugar, salt, and baking powder. Add milk and stir until there are no lumps.

4. Mix flour mixture in with melted butter (right into the skillet). Stir to mix thoroughly.

5. Slowly drop the fruit mixture on top of the flour batter. Do not stir in berries, just let them drop into the mixture as evenly as possible. Once you've dropped the berries in, don't touch it. Just put it in the oven for 35 – 40

minutes or until cooked through. (If the edges start to get brown simply cover with foil.)

Let cool for 10 minutes before eating. I know it's hard, but you don't want to burn your mouth. Add some ice cream and enjoy!

Note: IF there are any left overs, remove from pan and store in a different container. You never want to store food in cast iron as food can begin to take on a metallic flavor.

# Grain-Free Cookie Dough Truffles

*By Robin Konie*

**Ingredients:**

**For the cookie dough:**

1/2 cup almond butter

1/2 cup almond flour

1/4 cup grass-fed gelatin*

1/4 cup coconut oil, melted

1/4 cup butter, softened

1/2 tsp real salt

1/2 cup mini dark chocolate chips, fair trade please!

2 Tbs. organic maple syrup (grade B is best)

1 tsp vanilla extract

*Make sure you use the RIGHT kind of gelatin. Look for collagen hydrolysate. The brand I like is in a green can. This is the kind that won't gel.

**For the chocolate coating:**

1/2 cup dark chocolate chips

2 Tbsp. honey

2 Tbsp. coconut oil

1 tsp vanilla

**Directions:**

**For the cookie dough:**

1. Combine all ingredients except the chocolate chips in a mixing bowl. Stir until well combined. Then stir in the chocolate chips.

2. Scoop out small dough balls onto a cookie sheet (I love to use my handy cookie dough scooper for this). Chill in the refrigerator for 15 minutes.

3. Take slightly chilled dough balls out and mold them into perfect balls by gently rolling them between the palms of your hands. Place back in the fridge for thirty – sixty minutes.

**For the chocolate coating:**

1. Place all ingredients in a small sauce pan over low heat. Stir continuously until the chocolate is completely melted and everything is well combined. Turn heat off but leave the pan on the warm stove top.

**Assembling your truffles:**

1. Pull out your chilled dough balls. Drop one in the chocolate sauce and with two forks gently toss it around until it's fully covered. Tenderly scoop the ball up using the two forks and allow the excess chocolate drip off before transferring back to the cookie sheet.

2. Once all dough balls are covered, chill covered truffles in the fridge for another 15 – 30 minutes, or until the chocolate is well set.

Eat and enjoy now! Or, keep chilled to enjoy later. These truffles can be kept out at room temperature for an hour or two (hello, holiday parties!), but will keep better for longer time periods in the fridge.

## Cinnamon Maple Apple Crisp

*By Erica Hale*

**Ingredients:**

8 organic apples

1/3 cup organic cane sugar

2 tsp. organic ground cinnamon

1/2 tsp. organic ground nutmeg

**For topping:**

3 cups organic oats

1/2 cup organic raw butter, room temperature

1/2 cup organic cane sugar

1/2 cup organic maple syrup

3 tsp. cinnamon

1 tsp. nutmeg

1 tsp. organic vanilla extract

**Directions:**

1. Peel, core and slice the apples. Toss with the cane sugar, cinnamon and nutmeg and layer in an oven-safe baking dish.

2. Cream the butter. Add the oats, cane sugar, cinnamon and nutmeg. Slowly beat in the maple syrup and vanilla extract.

3. Crumble the topping over the apples.

4. Bake at 350 degrees, 25 minutes or until the apples are soft and the topping is browned around the edges.

5. Allow to cool for five minutes before serving.

## Cream Cheese Brownies

*By Robin Konie*

**Ingredients:**

**For the brownies:**

6 oz. chocolate chips, fair trade (I do 3 oz. each of dark and milk chocolate, but you can do whatever you like!)

1/2 cup (1 stick) of butter

3/4 cup rapadura sugar

1/2 tsp. pure vanilla extract

2 eggs

3/4 cup whole wheat or spelt flour (I choose either sprouted or freshly ground)

1/4 tsp real salt

**For the cream cheese top:**

1 8oz. package of organic cream cheese, room temperature

1/4 cup honey

1 egg

2 tsp pure vanilla extract

**Directions:**

Preheat oven to 350 degrees. Grease an 8×8″ glass baking dish.

For the brownies:

1. Cut butter into small cubes. In a small sauce pan, melt butter and chocolate chips over low heat, stirring consistently. Once completely melted remove from heat.

2. Stir in rapadura and vanilla with a large wooden spoon. Then add the eggs, 1 at a time, and stir vigorously until well combined.

3. Stir in flour and salt. Again, stir vigorously until well combined. Pour

brownie mixture into a well-greased baking dish.

For the cream cheese topping:

1. In a stand mixer, beat cream cheese until soft. Add the remaining ingredients and mix on medium-high until well combined.

2. Dollop cream cheese mixture on top of the brownie mixture. Spread with spatula and then drag a knife through the make swirls.

Bake for 30 – 35 minutes. Let cool on wire rack (like this). And then chill for a couple of hours before serving. (I promise, it's worth the wait!)

## Creamy Orange Zest Rice Pudding

*By Erica Hale*

**Ingredients for Stove Top:**

4 cups cooked organic white rice (1 1/2 cups dry rice, cooked until tender) *If using the slow cooker, 1 cup dry organic rice.

4 cups whole, organic raw milk (you can use coconut or almond milk) *If using the slow cooker, 8 cups milk or milk substitute.

3/4 cup organic evaporated cane sugar or Rapadura

2 cinnamon sticks

1/2 teaspoon ground nutmeg

1/2 cup organic raisins

2 teaspoons grated orange zest

1 teaspoon vanilla extract

2 organic, free range eggs (optional)

1/3 cup organic, raw heavy whipping cream (optional)

**Directions:**

1. Place cooked rice, milk, sugar, spices, raisins and orange zest in a large pot. Bring to a simmer, and continue to simmer (stirring frequently) for 20-25 minutes or until most of the liquid has been absorbed and the pudding is creamy. Or, if you're making this in the slow cooker, put the dry rice, milk, spices and orange zest into a buttered slow cooker (save the raisins for later). Set the slow cooker to low and allow to cook overnight (or 6-8 hours).

2. When the rice has absorbed most of the liquid, whisk the eggs, vanilla and cream together. Mix about a cup of the pudding into the egg mixture, then slowly add it to the rest of the pudding (to avoid having the eggs set…or, let your pudding cool a while before mixing in the eggs). If you'd like to make this vegan, you can omit this step…the pudding turns out fine without it!

3. If you're making the stove top version, cook and stir the pudding again until it's creamy and thick (5-7 minutes). If you're making it in the slow

cooker, add the raisins and turn the heat on the cooker up to high, allow it to cook another 30-45 minutes.

4. Serve hot, or chill for a few hours before serving. Store leftovers (if you have any!) in the fridge.

*Makes 6 large servings*

## Crème Brûlée

*By Robin Konie*

**Ingredients:**

2 cups cream (preferably raw)

6 egg yolks (preferably pastured)

1/2 cup pure maple syrup

1 tsp vanilla

A pinch of real salt

Sugar for topping (preferably Pure Organic Whole Cane Sugar)*

**Directions:**

1. Preheat oven to 300 degrees. Mix all ingredients together in a mixing bowl. (Don't whisk it!)

2. Strain custard mixture through a fine sieve

3. Pour into ramekins (depending on the size of ramekins it will probably fill 4 – 6. I usually get 5.)

4. Place ramekins into a 9 x 13″ glass baking dish. Fill baking dish with water so that it comes half way up the side of the ramekins.

5. Bake for 1 hour at 300 degrees, or until set. Let them cool at room temperature for 10 – 20 minutes and then transfer into the fridge. Chill for 2 hours – 3 days (as if they'll last that long!)

6. Just before serving, sprinkle 1/4 – 1/2 tsp of sugar on top of the crème brûlée and use a kitchen torch (or its likeness) to gently caramelize the sugar (you could also try putting it under the broiler, but watch it carefully!). Let it sit for five minutes before serving. (If using the whole sugar cane crystals, try grinding them up before adding on top.)

7. Devour!

*A note about the sugar on top:

What is the difference between "normal" sugar and Pure Organic Whole

Cane Sugar? Whole cane sugar, or Rapadura, is an unrefined sugar prized for its unique caramel flavor and fine grain texture. This deliciously pure sugar retains a beautiful golden color and offers unmatched nutritional value because – unlike other sugars – it is not separated from the molasses stream during squeeze-dried processing. This means there is some good stuff in there, like minerals. Awesome, right?

This sugar, because of its size, tends to burn more than caramelize when using a torch. I have found that putting the sugar in a bowl and then using the bottom of a cup to grind it up into a finer size makes it work wonderfully!

Of course you could always skip the "brûlée" part (crème brûlée means "burnt cream") and just eat the custard. It's delicious by itself, too.

## Double Chocolate Cookies

*By Robin Konie*

**Ingredients:**

1/2 cup sprouted wheat or spelt flour

1/3 cup unsweetened cocoa powder

3/4 tsp. cinnamon

1/2 tsp. baking aluminum free powder

1/2 tsp. baking soda

1/4 tsp. salt

1/3 cup sour cream (hint: low-fat and fat-free aren't real, okay?)

1/4 cup coconut oil

2/3 cup rapadura (organic whole cane sugar)

2 tsp. vanilla

1/4 cup dark chocolate chips (fair trade, please)

**Directions:**

Preheat oven to 350.

1. In a medium bowl or in your stand mixer, beat sour cream and coconut oil until well combined. Add in sugar and vanilla. Beat until combined.

2. On low, slowly mix in all the remaining ingredients except for the flour and chocolate chips. Mix until well combined.

3. Gently fold in flour and then the chocolate chips.

4. Place dough by the spoonful on a cookie sheet lined with parchment paper (I love my unbleached parchment paper for jobs like this). Flatten dough slightly either with your hand of the back of a spoon.

5. Bake at 350 for 10 minutes. Let cookies cool on sheet for another five before transferring to a wire rack.

*Makes 14 cookies*

## Gingerbread with Honey-Nutmeg Whipped Cream

*By Erica Hale*

**Ingredients:**

**Cake:**

1 1/2 cup organic wheat flour, OR 1 cup gluten free flour substitute, OR 1 cup almond flour and 1/2 cup coconut flour for grain free.

1/4 cup organic cane sugar

1/2 cup organic unsulphered blackstrap molasses

1/2 cup organic apples-only applesauce

2 Tablespoons raw butter, softened

1 large organic free range egg

1 Tablespoon freshly grated, organic ginger root

1 teaspoon ground cinnamon

1/2 teaspoon ground nutmeg

1/2 teaspoon ground clove

1/2 teaspoon non-aluminum baking powder

1/2 teaspoon baking soda

**Whipped Cream:**

2 cups organic, raw cream

1/3 cup raw honey

1 teaspoon ground nutmeg

**Directions:**

1. Preheat oven to 350 degrees, grease an 8×8 inch baking pan.

2. In a mixing bowl, combine all the ingredients for the cake and mix well.

3. Pour the batter into the greased pan, and bake for 35 to 40 minutes or until

a toothpick inserted in the center of the cake comes out clean.

4. Prepare the whipped cream: Beat the raw cream until it thickens. Once it begins to thicken, drizzle the honey into the bowl as you continue to beat the cream. When the whipped cream reaches the desired consistency, sprinkle in the nutmeg and beat a few seconds more, until combined.

5. Top the gingerbread with a generous dollop of whipped cream, and garnish with a touch of ground nutmeg.

*Serves 9*

# Grain-Free Birthday Cake

*By Robin Konie*

**Ingredients***

10 eggs, whisked

1 1/3 cup unsweetened organic applesauce

1/4 tsp strawberry liquid stevia

2/3 cup raw honey

2 Tbsp. vanilla extract

1 1/3 cup coconut flour, sifted

1 1/3 cup tapioca flour

1 1/2 cup almond flour

1/2 tsp real salt

1 tsp baking soda

1 tsp aluminum free baking powder

2/3 cup melted coconut oil

**Directions:**

1. Add all ingredients to a large mixing bowl

2. Mix using a stand mixer or hand mixer

3. Pour equal parts into 4 round 9 x 1.5 inch cake pans that have been greased.*

4. Bake at 325 degrees for 15 – 18 minutes, watching carefully the last few minutes to avoid over browning.

5. Let cool for five minutes and then transfer out of the pans onto a wire rack to cool completely

*You could easily half this recipe. As you can tell from my photos my cake was pretty tall and we had more than enough to go around for the 12 of us

there. If you half the recipe, just pour equal amounts of the batter into two cake pans instead of four.

I frosted my cake using a variation of this frosting recipe. Not sure I'd use it again, but it worked. Make sure to spread a very thin layer of frosting between the two layers to keep it from slipping. The real secret to making this cake yummy is to top it off with a simple strawberry compote. Delicious!

# Whole Orange Cake

*By Erica Hale*

**Ingredients:**

2 whole organic oranges, washed and chopped into large chunks

1 cup organic, raw butter

1 1/4 cups organic evaporated cane sugar or rapadura

3 large organic, free range eggs

2 1/2 cups organic, gluten free flour (or whole wheat flour, or your favorite flour blend)

1/2 teaspoon baking powder

1/4 teaspoon baking soda

**For Glaze:**

1 1/2 cups powdered organic cane sugar

2 Tablespoons plus 1 teaspoon organic orange juice, fresh squeezed

1 Tablespoon fresh orange zest

**Directions:**

1. Preheat oven to 325. Oil a 10 cup Bundt pan with coconut oil or raw butter, set aside. In a large bowl, beat together raw butter, cane sugar, and eggs.

2. Whirl orange chunks in a food processor until mostly smooth but not pureed, leaving some pieces of peel about the size of a current. Measure 1 1/2 cups of the oranges and add to the batter, beat until blended. Add the flour, baking powder and soda, and beat again until smooth. Spread the batter into the prepared pan.

3. Bake for 55 minutes, or until a toothpick inserted into the cake comes out with just a few crumbs on it. Cool for 10 minutes, then invert the cake onto a plate and allow it to cook completely (do let it cool all the way…we rushed this step and the glaze melted into the cake. Tastes good, but not as pretty!)

4. Prepare the glaze: Mix the sugar, orange juice and zest together in a bowl. Pour over the cooled cake.

Enjoy!

# Homemade Peppermint Patties

*By Robin Konie*

**Ingredients:**

For peppermint filling:

1 ¾ cup powdered sugar

¾ - 1 cup coconut oil

¼ tsp real salt

1 tsp peppermint extract

For chocolate coating:

8 oz. dark chocolate chips (fair trade, please)

2 tsp coconut oil

**Directions:**

1. Mix all the peppermint filling ingredients together in a medium bowl. Use the back of a spoon to "cream" together the ingredients. Start with just 1/2 cup of coconut oil and add in up to one cup until you get a nice firm consistency that sticks together when you squeeze it.

2. Form mixture into small discs and place on a baking sheet lined with waxed paper. Place in freezer for about 10 minutes while you make the chocolate coating.

3. Heat chocolate and 2 tsp of coconut oil in a medium saucepan over medium-low heat. Stir continuously to avoid scorching. Remove from heat once fully melted.

4. Drop discs into chocolate. Using a small spoon turn over a couple of times to completely cover. Take out with a fork and let the excess chocolate drip off before moving them back to the lined baking sheet.

5. Place covered discs back in the freezer and keep there until firm. Store in fridge or freezer to prevent melting.

Note: I used homemade powdered sugar made from Rapadura. This gives a light brown color to the peppermint filling. But it still tastes delicious!

Enjoy!

# Homemade Powdered Sugar

*By Robin Konie*

**Ingredients:**

1 cup sweetener of your choice, like Rapadura

1 Tbsp. arrowroot powder

**Directions:**

Put ingredients in a blender. Blend until a consistent powder is formed.

## Raw Homemade Vanilla Ice Cream

*By Robin Konie*

**Ingredients:**

3 1/2 cups of raw organic cream (any cream will do, but raw gives you extra healthy benefits if you can get your hands on it).

4 pastured egg yolks

1/2 cup organic cane sugar or organic maple syrup

2 tbsp. pure vanilla extract

1 tbsp. raw honey

A generous pinch of real sea salt

**Directions:**

1. Beat the eggs yolks in a medium size bowl
2. Add the remaining ingredients and whisk to combine.
3. Pour into ice cream maker and follow manufacturer's directions.

Enjoy it in its out-of-the-ice-cream-maker-softy-goodness, or place in an air tight container with plastic wrap over the ice cream to consume later.

*You can add strawberries, chocolate chips, or any other topping. Just add for the last couple of minutes of churning.

## Pear Upside Down Cake with Honey Ginger Sauce

*By Erica Hale*

**Ingredients:**

**Cake:**

2 Tbsp. organic raw butter

1/4 cup raw honey

1 Tbsp. organic lemon juice

3 organic pears, cored and thinly sliced

1 cup organic cane sugar

2 eggs

1/2 cup organic applesauce

1 cup organic, unbleached flour (or, 1 cup gluten free flour substitute, or use 1/2 cup almond flour mixed with 1/2 cup coconut flour for grain-free)

**Honey-Ginger Sauce:**

2 Tbsp. organic raw butter

1/4 cup raw honey

1 Tbsp. freshly grated organic ginger root

2 Tbsp. organic lemon juice

**Directions:**

Preheat oven to 350

**Cake:**

1. Melt butter in a large skillet, add honey and lemon juice.

2. Add sliced pears, simmer until the pears are transparent and soft (7-10 minutes).

3. In a bowl, combine the sugar, flour, eggs, and applesauce.

4. Remove the pears from the skillet and arrange the slices in the bottom of a

greased 9 inch round pan, leaving the liquid in the skillet.

5. Pour the cake batter over the sliced pears, and bake at 350 for 35 minutes (or until a toothpick inserted in the center comes out clean).

6. Allow the cake to cool for 15 minutes, then slide a knife around the edges to loosen. Invert the cake on a platter.

**Honey-Ginger Sauce:**

1. Add the butter, honey, lemon juice and ginger to the skillet that the pears simmered in (add to the liquid left over).

2. Simmer the sauce until it begins to thicken, remove from heat and set aside.

Serve the upside down cake with the sauce drizzled on top.

## Honey Sweetened Strawberry Lemon Sorbet

*By Robin Konie*

**Ingredients:**

16 oz. organic strawberries (about 2 – 3 cups)

Juice of 3 organic lemons

Zest of 1 lemon

1/4 cup of raw honey

3 -4 dashes of real sea salt

**Directions:**

1. Pour lemon juice, zest, and strawberries into food processor or blender. Blend until well combined.

2. Add honey one tablespoon at a time, mix, and taste. Continue to add until it's at your desired sweetness. Add salt. Blend until well combined.

3. Put in refrigerator until well chilled.

4. Pour mixture into your ice cream maker and churn according to manufacturer's directions.*

5. Scoop into an air tight container and freeze for 2 hours before serving. (Confession: I usually don't do this last step. A soft sorbet is just my thing.)

*If you don't have an ice cream make your can just freeze the blended mixture in an air tight container. It won't be quite as smooth, but it will still taste good.

# Sprouted Banana Bread Recipe

*By Robin Konie*

**Ingredients:**

2 cups sprouted whole wheat flour

3/4 cup organic whole cane sugar

1/2 tsp baking soda

1/2 tsp salt

1 tsp ground cinnamon

3 ripe bananas, smashed

2 large eggs, beaten

6 tbsp. butter, melted

1 tsp vanilla

1/4 cup plain yogurt (recipe to make your own found here.)

**Directions:**

Preheat oven to 350. Butter and flour a bread pan.

1. In a bowl, combine flour, sugar, baking soda, salt, and cinnamon. Mix thoroughly.

2. In a separate bowl, combined smashed bananas, eggs, melted butter, vanilla, and yogurt.

3. Gently fold dry ingredients into wet ingredients (be careful not to over "smash" your banana bits). Scoop into prepared bread pan. Dough will be thick. Use a spatula to even it out in the pan.

4. Bake for 40 – 50 minutes in a 350 degree oven. (Oven times will vary, check at 35 minutes and continue baking until a toothpick comes out clean.) Let cool in pan for 10 minutes and then move to wire rack to cool completely.

# Sprouted Chocolate Chip Cookie

*By Robin Konie*

**Ingredients:**

2 cups sprouted whole wheat (or spelt) flour

1 tsp baking soda

1 tsp real salt

1/2 cup coconut oil (melted)

1/2 cup butter (softened, preferably pastured and raw)

1 cup natural rapadura

2 tsp vanilla extract

2 eggs (preferably pastured)

1 cup of dark chocolate chips (fair trade, please)

**Directions:**

Preheat Oven to 350 degrees.

1. Cream sugar, butter, and coconut oil until smooth
2. Add in eggs and vanilla, mix on low until incorporated
3. Still on low speed, mix in salt and baking soda
4. Stir in flour by hand
5. Stir in chips by hand

Scoop dough out by the spoon full on a greased baking sheet. Bake for 8 – 9 minutes. Let cool on pan for 5 minutes then transfer to wire rack to cool completely.

Enjoy!

## Stuffed Baked Apples

*By Erica Hale*

**Ingredients:**

**For each apple:**

1 fresh, organic apple (Fuji, Gala and Honeycrisp work well)

1/2 tablespoon raw, organic butter

1 tablespoon organic raisins

1 tablespoon organic dried apricots

1 tablespoon organic dried cranberries

1 tablespoon organic rolled oats

1 tablespoon organic grade B maple syrup

Optional: Experiment with chopped nuts, shredded coconut, flax seed, dried blueberries or chopped dates.

**For topping:**

1/4 cup raw whipping cream

1 tablespoon raw, organic honey

(This makes enough topping to very generously top one apple, doubling it will top 4.)

**Directions:**

1. Wash, core and slice your apples. You can use an apple slicer/corer, leave the apple in the corer and tie it back together with kitchen twine. Carefully wiggle the core out of the apple and remove the apple from the corer. Place it in a glass baking dish (if you're doing more than one, pack them in together so that they hold each other up). Or, you can just core the apples.

2. In a bowl, mix the butter, dried fruit, maple syrup, and oats.

3. Stuff the apples with the fruit and oat mixture, there may be extra that can be piled on top of the apple or baked in the dish next to the apples.

4. Bake the apples at 325 degrees for 40 minutes (or until they are soft).

5. Whip the cream until it becomes thick and frothy. Drizzle the honey into the cream as it's being whipped, right before serving.

6. Serve the apples with a dollop of whipped cream. Remove the string and let the apples fall, then eat like an apple crisp.

## Sweet Summer Berry Cobbler

*By Robin Konie*

**Ingredients:**

**Crumble Top:**

1/3 cup sprouted wheat or spelt flour

3/4 cup rolled oats

1/2 cup nuts (we like walnuts and almonds together)

3 Tbs butter or coconut oil

1/4 cup raw honey or organic maple syrup (grade B)

**Berry Filling:**

1/4 cup raw honey

2 tsp cinnamon

2 -3 lbs. of fresh berries (organic is best if you got them) OR 2 10 – 14 oz. bags of frozen berries (cut any large berries into bite-size pieces).

**Directions:**

Preheat oven to 350°

1. In a food processor or blender, combine all the crumble top ingredients. Blend well and set aside.

2. In a bowl, combine honey and cinnamon. Add fruit and stir well to coat. Put filling in a lightly oiled 8 x 8" baking pan or pie plate.

3. Crumble topping ingredients over the top.

4. Bake for 20 – 30 minutes or until fruit is tender and topping is browned.

**Tip**: If top starts browning too soon, loosely cover with foil while fruit continues to bake.

I love to cut the recipe in half and make individual servings in small ramekins. That way there isn't too many left-overs to tempt me the rest of the night!

Cool and enjoy!

*Serves 4*

# Whipped Coconut Cream

*By Erica Hale*

**Ingredients:**

1 can organic coconut milk

1-3 tablespoons organic evaporated cane sugar, sucanat, raw honey or maple syrup

1/2 teaspoon organic vanilla (optional)

**Directions:**

1. Chill the can of coconut milk for at least an hour. If it's hot out, also chill the bowl you'll be using to whip the cream.

2. Separate the hardened coconut cream from the liquid in the can. The easiest way to do this is to flip the can upside down and open it that way, then pour off the liquid before scooping out the "cream".

3. Whip the coconut cream on high speed with your mixer. Slowly add the sweetener of your choice…if you're using honey or maple syrup, you'll want to drizzle it in a very small amount at a time. The coconut cream is naturally a little sweet, so start with a little sweetener and taste it to see when you're happy with the flavor. If you're adding the vanilla, add it now as well.

4. Continue to whip the coconut mixture until it is thick. Don't over mix, as it will melt if it gets too warm!

5. Serve right away, and keep any unused portion in the fridge. If it's been refrigerated for a while and is very cold, it will harden. Just whip it again for a second before you serve it!

# DRESSINGS, CONDIMENTS, & PANTRY STAPLES

## Homemade Butter and Buttermilk

*By Robin Konie*

**Ingredients:**

Cream (any amount, but the more you have the more butter you get)

Ice water (optional, but it does help preserve the butter longer)

Salt (optional, but again, helps the butter "keep" longer)

**Directions:**

1. Place cream in your blender or food processor. Making sure the lid is tight, start blending on high for 5 – 10 minutes. Ultimately you are taking your cream well beyond the "whipped cream" phase into an almost curdled phase.

2. Once your cream is well curdled and you see the fat start to separate from the milk, let it rest for a couple of minutes.

3. Pour the contents of the blender/processor into a cheesecloth (I've used a flour cloth, too). Squeeze out all the liquid into a bowl. Congratulations! That is your buttermilk!

4. Dump the butter that is left in the cheesecloth back into the food processor and pour some ice water over the butter. You don't need a lot, just enough to help "rinse" the butter from any remaining buttermilk. This is technically an "optional" step but it will help your butter last longer.

5. Pulse your blender/processor a couple of times.

7. Pour contents back into cheesecloth. Squeeze out (and discard) remaining water. Congratulations! What's left in your cheesecloth is butter. Feel free to add some sea salt or other herbs to make salted butter, herb butter, etc.

8. Pat yourself on the back. You are officially old school.

# Homemade Mayonnaise

*By Erica Hale*

**Ingredients:**

2 organic, free range eggs

2 Tablespoons organic apple cider vinegar with the Mother

1/2 Teaspoon organic powdered mustard

1/2 Teaspoon sea salt

2 cups organic, cold pressed extra-virgin olive oil

**Directions:**

1. In a food processor, blend eggs, apple cider vinegar, mustard and sea salt. Pulse until combined.

2. With the food processor going, slowly drizzle the oil into the egg mixture. You need to do this slowly, make sure that only a thin stream of oil is going in. If you're doing it right, you will probably have to set the measuring cup down at least once because your arm will get tired!

3. Continue to run the food processor until the mayonnaise thickens. If your mayo isn't thick enough, add a little more oil and process it longer.

4. Spoon the mayonnaise into a canning jar, secure the lid and store it in the fridge for up to two weeks.

# Dressed up Mayonnaise (3 Ways)

*By Erica Hale*

**Ingredients:**

**For Basil and Sun Dried Tomato:**

1/2 cup mayonnaise (all natural or homemade)

2 tablespoons chopped organic sun dried tomatoes

1 tablespoon chopped organic basil (I used Opal Basil)

1 clove organic garlic, pressed

Sea salt to taste

**For Jalapeno Chili:**

1/2 cup mayonnaise (all natural or homemade)

2 tablespoons finely diced organic jalapeno

2 teaspoons organic lime juice

1 teaspoon organic chili powder

**For Garlic Aioli:**

1/2 cup mayonnaise (all natural or homemade)

3 cloves organic garlic, pressed

2 teaspoons organic lemon juice

Sea salt to taste

Organic cracked black pepper to taste

**Directions:**

1. Choose and prepare your ingredients.
2. Mix them together with the mayonnaise.
3. Cover and refrigerate for at least an hour (overnight is best) before serving, to allow the flavors to diffuse.

4. Store in the fridge in an airtight container, for up to one week.

## Homemade Yogurt

*By Erica Hale*

**Ingredients:**

If you are using grass-fed, organic pasteurized/homogenized milk:

2 quarts milk (organic, grass-fed pasteurized, homogenized)

1/4 to 1/2 cup yogurt starter (you can use plain organic yogurt with live cultures from the store, or use yogurt from a previous batch you made at home)

If you are using organic, grass-fed raw milk:

2 quarts raw milk (the fresher, the better!)

1/2 teaspoon freeze-dried yogurt starter, or 1/2 cup store-bought organic plain yogurt from the store

**Directions:**

**For pasteurized/homogenized milk:**

Measure 2 quarts of milk, pour it into a large pot. Bring milk to 185 degrees, using a kitchen thermometer to monitor the heat (for thicker yogurt, you can let it sit at 185 degrees for 10-20 minutes before turning down the heat). Turn off the heat under the milk, and let it cool to 110 degrees. Once milk is 110 degrees, add the yogurt starter and stir well. Pour into 2 quart sized canning jars, put on the lids, and place in your oven. Turn the oven light on, close the door and leave overnight or for 9-12 hours.

In the morning, remove the yogurt from the oven and store it in the fridge.

**For raw milk:**

Measure out 2 quarts of milk as described above. Heat milk to 110 degrees, using a kitchen thermometer to monitor the heat. Mix in the powdered yogurt starter or store-bought yogurt. Pour milk into quart jars, put on the lid and leave in your oven overnight with the light on, as described above.

In the morning, stir the yogurt well. If you would like thicker yogurt, strain it by pouring it into a layered piece of cheesecloth. Wrap the cheesecloth around the yogurt and gently twist until the whey drips out (you can use this to culture vegetables, etc. so save it for later!). Tie the cheesecloth up at the top and place it in a sieve, then place the sieve in a bowl and put the whole thing in the fridge for a few hours. Once the whey has drained off, put the thickened yogurt back into the jars and return it to the fridge.

# Lacto-Fermented Green Tomato Salsa

*By Erica Hale*

**Ingredients:**

About 6 medium sized, organic green tomatoes…or a combination of smaller tomatoes to make about 4 or 5 cups of chopped tomatoes.

1 or 2 organic red tomatoes

5 organic red jalapenos

2 organic green banana peppers

1 large organic onion

1/2 cup organic cilantro (optional)

7 cloves organic garlic

3 tablespoons organic fresh lemon juice

2 tablespoons kombucha or organic apple cider vinegar with "The Mother"

1 teaspoon raw organic yogurt with active cultures

3 teaspoons sea salt

3 teaspoons all-natural chili powder

**Directions:**

1. Run the fresh tomatoes, onion and peppers through a food processor (I use the shredding attachment), or chop them finely by hand. Put them all in a large mixing bowl.

2. Crush or mince the garlic. Mince the cilantro, and add them both to the tomato mixture.

3. Stir in the lemon juice, apple cider vinegar or kombucha. Add yogurt and chili powder and salt and stir well.

4. Pack salsa in sterilized jars, using a canning funnel. Top with fermentation lids and firmly tighten the lids down on the jars. Fill fermentation bubblers with water.

5. Set aside for 3 days to 2 weeks (checking the taste periodically) in a cool, dark place away from sunlight.

6. After fermentation, remove the fermentation lids and replace with regular canning lids. You can process the jars for 30 minutes in hot water and store, or just put them in cold storage. Processing with hot water will result in the live cultures being killed, so mine are going in the fridge!

# Parmesan Ranch Dressing

*By Robin Konie*

**Ingredients:**

2 cups plain yogurt (full fat, please!)

1 tbsp. mayonnaise (homemade or find one that's made with only quality olive oil)

1/4 cup finely chopped green onions

2 tbsp. dried parsley

1/2 tsp real salt

1/4 cup Parmesan cheese, finely grated

(2 tabs milk, optional)

**Directions:**

1. Combine all ingredients (except the milk) in a small bowl.

2. Taste and add more salt or cheese as needed.

3. If you prefer a thinner dressing, slowly add in milk, 1 tablespoon at a time until you get your desired thickness. (I prefer mine without the milk.)

## Honey Mustard Poppy Seed Dressing

*By Robin Konie*

**Ingredients:**

½ c. Whole grain mustard

½ c. Dijon mustard

3 Tbs. Honey

1 tsp. Apple Cider Vinegar (Raw, Organic is best…)

1 tsp Extra Virgin Olive Oil

1 – 2 tbsp. poppy seeds

**Directions:**

1. In a small bowl mix mustards together with a fork. Stir in honey and vinegar.

2. Whisk in Olive Oil until fully incorporated

3. Stir in poppy seeds.

From here you can move this over into some sort of "dressing" container. But I won't judge you if you just keep it in the same bowl. I'm all about doing less dishes.

## Yogurt Cream Cheese

*By Erica Hale*

**Ingredients:**

12-16 ounces fresh yogurt of your choice (I use homemade)

**You will need:**

Cheesecloth

Strainer

Large Jar, pitcher or deep bowl

Kitchen twine

**Directions:**

1. Layer 3 pieces of cheesecloth in a strainer. Set the strainer in a deep plate, and spoon your yogurt onto the cloth. The plate will catch the liquid as it starts to drip out.

2. Fold the cloth around the cheese, and tightly tie it at the top to form a ball. Tie this ball to a long spoon, and hang it in a large jar, pitcher or deep bowl. Place the whole thing in your fridge, and leave it for 24 hours.

3. Line a small container of your choice with several layers of cheesecloth. Press the cheese into the container, folding the top of the cloth over the cheese. Place plastic wrap on top of the cloth, then cut a circle of cardboard to rest on top of the cheese. Place a heavy object (I use a canning jar filled with water) on top of the cardboard, and return to the fridge for 2-3 days.

4. Carefully un-mold the cheese, turning it onto a serving plate and removing the cloth. Serve plain, or with a topping (like roasted garlic and chives, or drizzle with honey and sprinkle with crushed pistachios and serve with apples as a dessert).

Store any unused cheese in the fridge.

# BEVERAGES

# All Natural Italian Cream Soda

*By Erica Hale*

**Ingredients:**

4 cups organic, 100% fruit juice (pomegranate, blueberry and cherry are great!)

2 cups organic raw cream

1/4 cup organic cane sugar

2 bottles natural sparkling mineral water

**Directions:**

1. Pour the 4 cups of juice into a sauce pan and bring to a boil over high heat. Reduce heat to medium-low and simmer juice for 60-80 minutes, until it has reduced to a thick syrup. The time it will need to simmer varies depending on the natural sugar content of the juice, so plan ahead on this step and keep an eye on the stove!

2. Allow the syrup to cool for at least 2o minutes.

3. While the syrup cools, whip raw, organic cream with the cane sugar until it's thick and frothy.

4. Pour about 10 ounces of sparkling mineral water into a glass, followed by 2 or 3 tablespoons of the fruit juice syrup and 1 tablespoon of cream.

5. Add ice cubes to taste.

5. Top with as much whipped cream as you can handle!

Store left over fruit juice syrup in the fridge for the next round of soda.

# Holiday Eggnog

*By Erica Hale*

**Ingredients:**

4 large free range, organic eggs

2 cups organic raw milk

1 cup organic raw cream

1/3 cup plus 1 tablespoon organic cane sugar or Rapadura

1 teaspoon organic pure vanilla extract

1/2 teaspoon freshly ground nutmeg

1/4 teaspoon ground cinnamon

Dash ground cloves

**Directions:**

1. Separate the eggs, and set the whites aside. In a large bowl, beat the yolks with 1/3 cup sugar until they are thick and lighter in color. This may take a while!

2. If you are heating your milk, pour the milk and cream into a saucepan and heat on the stove until it just begins to steam. If you're leaving the milk raw, skip this step and move on to the next!

3. Add the spices and vanilla to the cream and milk mixture.

4. If you heated the milk, combine 1 cup of the hot milk with the egg yolk mixture while stirring. Whisk for a minute or so, then combine the rest of the milk with the yolk mixture. If you're leaving it raw, just combine the milk with the yolks.

5. In a different bowl, whip the egg whites and the 1 Tablespoon of sugar until they stiff peaks form.

6. Gently fold the whipped egg whites into the eggnog, and stir until combined.

7. Chill and serve!

## Zesty Homemade Vegetable Juice Cocktail

*By Erica Hale*

**Ingredients:**

9 organic tomatoes (roma work well)

4 stalks organic celery (leaves included)

7 large organic carrots

1 cup organic parsley

1 organic green bell pepper, quartered (leave the seeds in)

1-2 cloves organic garlic, according to taste

1/4 organic red onion

1/2 organic beet

7 organic radishes

1/4 inch wide slice of organic horseradish root (or adjust to taste)

1/2 to 1 teaspoon cayenne pepper (adjust to taste)

2 tsp organic apple cider vinegar

**Directions:**

1. Wash all the vegetables well.

2. Run them through a juicer according to your juicers instructions, into a large bowl or container.

3. Once all the vegetables have been juiced, mix in the pepper and vinegar well. Serve right away. It's fun to garnish this with small stalks of celery!

4. Drink right away, or store for up to 8 hours in the fridge.

*Yields 4-6 servings of juice*

www.ingramcontent.com/pod-product-compliance
Lightning Source LLC
LaVergne TN
LVHW041104150826
845673LV00007B/1910

*9798473181135*